Critical Actions to Change Your Life
A Workbook for a New You

How Your Attitude Brings You Suffering or Peace

Jane E Perri, PhD, DHT

Southern Ohio Press
Dayton Ohio

Copyright © 2015 Jane E. Perri

All rights reserved. No part of this book may be used or reproduced by any means, graphic, electronic, or mechanical, including photocopying, recording, taping or by any information storage retrieval system without the written permission of the publisher except in the case of brief quotations embodied in critical articles and reviews.

Southern Ohio Press books may be ordered through booksellers or by contacting:

Southern Ohio Press
617 Kling Drive
Dayton, Ohio 45416
www.SouthernOhioPress.com
937-750-5416

Because of the dynamic nature of the Internet, any web addresses or links contained in this book may have changed since publication and may no longer be valid. The views expressed in this work are solely those of the author and do not necessarily reflect the views of the publisher, and the publisher hereby disclaims any responsibility for them.

ISBN: 978-0-9964693-0-2 (sc)

Printed in the United States of America.

Book cover design and illustration by Danny Mangelsdorf.

Dedication

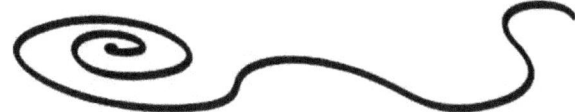

This book is dedicated to all my children and children-in-law (Taylor, Philip, Rowena, Amanda, Tricia, Ellie, and Charles) and grandchildren (Gino, Adriana, Nicolas, Emma, Piper, and any others who may come along). May travel on your path in life be easier than those of us who have gone before you. You will not be able to avoid the pain of life but you can avoid the suffering. May your lives be filled with joy, peace, and contentment for all that you have and all that you have not. I love you all.

Acknowledgments

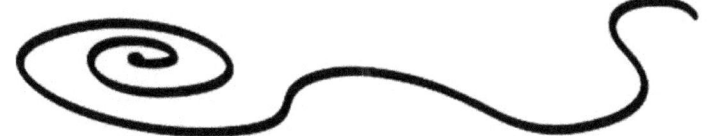

I wish to thank the members of the Dharma Center of Dayton sangha for their support in writing this workbook. Their feedback on the philosophy and exercises was extremely helpful. I also wish to thank Marye Hefty (author of *Madeline's Prayer*), Marilyn Cranbil, and Carol Johnson who kept after me to "just get it done." The manuscript would probably still be sitting in the digital void without their push. Thank you Marilyn, Carol, and Sallie Ortiz for taking your precious time to edit the copy of the book. It certainly reads more smoothly with your voices.

Danny Mangelsdorf is the creator of the wonderful painting of a quilted spiral. The original art is 35" x 35" and is hanging in the Dharma Center of Dayton. With one simple idea, he captured the true meaning of this message. Thank you so much Danny for your vision.

Thank you to all my teachers over the years. Truly this book is the sum total of what I have learned from all of you. A special appreciation to the two buddhas who shared their wisdom, gave me direction, and changed my life. This book would not exist if not for you both. Thank you for giving me the opportunity to share your medicine with the world.

Finally, thanks to my loving husband Paul Oswald for putting up with the process for the last several years, your patience and understanding is very much appreciated. I love you.

Contents

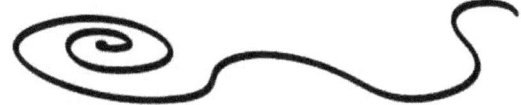

Dedication iii

Acknowledgments v

Note to Reader xi

Preface xiii

Part One: Philosophy
Theory of the Universal Spiral of Love 1

Ego Traits: Four Basic States of Human Ego Emotions 3
1 Release of Anger 3
2 Release of Fear 5
3 Release of Prejudice 6
4 Release of Separation 8

Spiritual Traits: Three Higher States of Spiritual Essences 11
5 Acknowledging Acceptance 11
6 Acknowledging Compassion 13
7 Acknowledging Love 15

Between the Lines and the Core of the Spiral 19
8 Between the Layers—Ego and Grace 19
9 Core of the Spiral—Trust 19
10 Spirals as Symbols 21
11 How to Use the Spiral for Personal Growth and Healing 22
12 Conclusion 24

Part Two: Practice
Reflective Readings to Illustrate Each Layer of the Spiral 29

13 Release of Anger 29

  Picking Weeds 29
  Societal Anger 32
  Getting Even 35
  Painters' Pants 37

14 Release of Fear 40
  Prevailing Winds 40
  Setting boundaries 43
  Is Competition Healthy? 44
  Overcoming Fear 47

15 Release of Prejudice 49
  Life is Easy 49
  School Days Traumas 51
  Prejudging Our Neighbors 54

16 Release of Separation 56
  Which Religion Gets it Right? 57
  Dance for Your Life 59
  The Value of One Life 62
  Abandonment 64
  War Mindset 65
  Garage Sales 66

17 Acknowledging Acceptance 70
  Bone Spurs 70
  Happy Birthday 73

18 Acknowledging Compassion 74
  Ego Control and Finding Your Way 74
  On Wealth, Fame, and the Pursuit of a Really Great Loaf of Bread 76
  The Price is Right 77
  Stop Trying to Do Good 78

19 Acknowledging Love 82
  Gift of Life 82
  Love: Conventional and Otherwise 84
  Friendship Today 84
  Charity—the Gift of Love to Yourself 85

20 Spaces Between the Lines—Ego and Grace 90
  Life is Like a Box of Chocolates 90

21 The Core—Trust 93
  Trusting Your Instincts 93
  Unfinished Objects 95
  The Glue that Holds Relationships Together—Trust 96

Part Three: Additional Practices
   Reflective Readings to Illustrate Other Critical Practices 103

22 Attachment 103
   Forgotten Existence 104
   Crying 104
   Asleep Standing 106
   Changing Old Floor Coverings 107

23 Peace 110
   What is Peace? 110
   Wanting Peace and Getting It 111

24 Healthy Behaviors 111
   The Center of All Life 111
   Where Did the Wild Ones Go? 113
   Free Will 114
   Healthy Living 116
   Thanksgiving Day—The Point of Giving Thanks 118
   Depression 118
   All Red Roses 120
   It's All a Game 121
   Ring of Fire 123
   Mudra—Have No Fear 124
   Living Life Easy 126
   It is Not Summertime Everywhere 131
   Show and Shine Drive-In 133
   Moving into a New Home 134
   Coffee, Tea, or Me or Ten Steps to a Better You 135
   Bicycling in the Snow 137
   Is Truth Situational? 143
   Sticking to Something that Matters 144
   What is the Purpose of Life? 150
   Be the Wave of Compassion 152
   To Be Reborn 154
   The Ending is the Beginning 157

Exercises
1. Forgiveness Part I 30
2. Forgiveness Part II 33
3. Forgiveness Part III 35
4. Mirror, Mirror on the Wall 38
5. Assess Your Relationships 42
6. Examine Your Fears 46
7. Mindful Breathing 48
8. Self-Examination I 53
9. Reach Out 55

10.	All the Same	58
11.	Ask or Tell	60
12.	Value of Life	63
13.	Ethical Guidelines	68
14.	Self-Examination II	71
15.	Self-Examination Meditation	73
16.	Good Bread Recipe	76
17.	Good Deeds Without Intent	79
18.	Who Helped You?	87
19.	Chocolate Sensation	91
20.	UFO Day	96
21.	Trust	97
22.	Getting Control of Your Pain	105
23.	Practice of Being	113
24.	Living a Fulfilling Life	117
25.	Have No Fear	125
26.	Replacing Attachment with Gratitude	128
27.	Palpable Emotional Output	132
28.	Ten Steps to a Better You	136
29.	Developing your Spiritual Practice	140
30.	Develop Your Personal Mission, Vision, and Values Statements	144
31.	Power to Change	153
32.	The New Me	155

Glossary 159

Bibliography 165

About the Author 167

Note to the Reader

The inspiration for this book came from a series of conversations with two spiritual mentors that offered their voices to try to help heal and calm the terrible chaos that the world is embroiled in today. They have asked that they not be identified directly because they believe that the concepts are so universal that they should not be claimed by any one person. In fact, the information has been given to many different people with the hope that at least one or two will put the ideas into writing and spread the message far and wide. With that intention, this wonderful message of hope, liberation from suffering, and joy is brought to you in this book.

Please share it with all you know. Humanity is not doomed to live in mental, emotional, and spiritual suffering. This text will give you seven basic ideas that you can use to improve not only your life but also the lives of all those you touch. Please accept this gift from the hearts of those who have found their bliss through the adoption of these attitude and behaviors.

I am blessed to be one of the fortunate people with whom this message of hope has been shared. It is my great pleasure to pass it on to you.

Preface

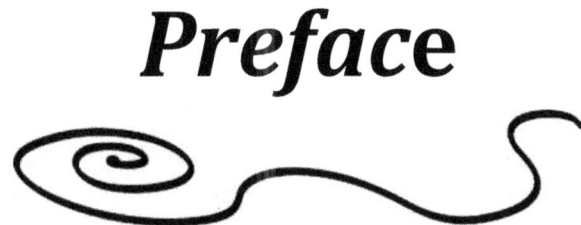

Our attitudes influence how we see the world, how we see ourselves, and how we view all situations in which we find ourselves. If we consider our lives to be full of suffering, then they are. If we say that the world is not fair to us, then it's not. The mind is an extremely powerful tool to change our very existence by simply changing our thoughts. Repeated thoughts in a single vein, ultimately becomes the architecture of our lives.

A Buddhist teaching says, "Pain is inevitable, suffering is optional." Pain refers to the physical pain of injury, sickness, and physical decay of our bodies, which happens as we move through life toward death. Suffering refers to our mental, emotional, and spiritual response to pain, to our relationships, to our jobs, and to all of life's events. We have little if any control over our pain, but we are in complete control of our suffering. It is suffering and its elimination that is the topic of this text. When you change your attitude toward your pain, you eliminate your suffering.

There are seven actions that, if mastered, will eliminate suffering in your life. Our attitude is the engine that drives our ability to take these actions. Those seven actions are represented by a spiral, each layer of the spiral representing a different mental state. This spiral is called the—"The Universal Symbol of Love."

The theory is that each layer of the spiral represents one of the four basic ego states of human emotion or one of three higher states of our spiritual essence. The innermost layer represents the release of anger that is entrenched within us. The next layers of the spiral are, in order, release of fear, release of prejudice, release of separation, acknowledgment of acceptance, acknowledgment of compassion, and acknowledgment of love. At the core of the spiral is trust.

The potent physical impact of negative emotion on the human body has been widely studied and confirmed. The emotions of anger, fear, and prejudice are obviously destructive in their nature. Separation, as interpreted in Buddhist thought, sheds light on why the philosophy of individualism is damaging to our mental and spiritual health.

The last three layers of the spiral are tools for curing disease brought about by the first four layers of anger, fear, prejudice, and separation. However, without acknowledging our ego's desires to control, not only ourselves, but others and our environment, it is impossible to use these tools.

The book is divided in three parts: philosophy, practice of the states of the spiral and other important practices. Each layer of the spiral is discussed in the philosophy section and then illustrated by stories in the first practice section. The stories are individual stand-alone readings and the seed for group discussion. Most of the stories have associated exercises to help you better understand yourself and why you do what you do.

The Tools

Four Basic States of Human Ego Emotion	T R U S T	Three Higher States of Spiritual Essence
1 Release of anger		5 Acknowledgement of acceptance
2 Release of fear		6 Acknowledgement of compassion
3 Release of prejudice		7 Acknowledgement of love
4 Release of separation		

Part One: Philosophy

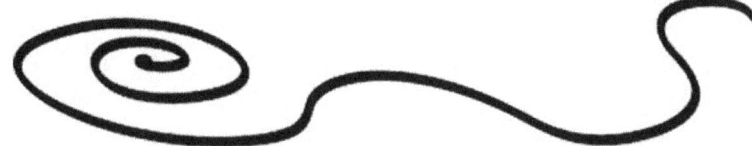

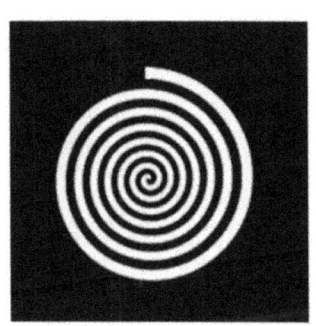

Part One: Philosophy

Theory of the Universal Spiral of Love

In the beginning of time, there was nothing but energy and simple matter, everything was connected. Scientists theorize that the universe began as a result of a "Big Bang." The original hypothesis is attributed to Belgian cosmologist and Catholic priest Georges Lemaître. He suggested the Big Bang theory in the 1920s and published it in scientific literature in 1931. The theory stated that a small group of tightly compacted particles exploded and traveled in all directions. This was the early genesis of the stars and planets, hence the universe was born.
(science.nationalgeographic.com/science/space/universe/origins-universe-article)

Current theory has altered this version of what happened slightly but in a dramatically important way. Instead of the pieces separating, they stayed together in something that resembles a spider web. All the pieces remained connected with no separation between them and all continue to remain connected today. Aerospace computer systems designer, Gregg Braden calls the container that holds the universe "The Divine Matrix." He says that this matrix "is the bridge between all things, and the mirror that shows us what we have created" (Braden 4). Braden writes in his book titled *Divine Matrix* that "to tap the force of the universe itself, we must see ourselves as part of the world rather than separate from it" (Braden 11).

In *The Divine Matrix,* Braden provides scientific support for this eternal connection through the discussion of numerous replicated physics studies. By investigating proton mirroring and holograms, scientists have shown that "in a holographic 'something,' every piece of the something mirrors the whole something.... The universally connected hologram of consciousness promises that the instant we create our good wishes and prayers, they are already received at their destination.... [Therefore] through the hologram of consciousnesses, a little change in our lives is mirrored everywhere in our world" (Braden 103).

Most people in the world tend to believe that people are distinct, disconnected, and unrelated other than through family lines. Some cultures are more group, family, or cluster-oriented while others are more individualistic. The United States is strongly individualistic and the "family" is typically composed of the parents and children. Extended family members may play a role but not necessarily a strong one. Collective cultures view their entire extended family as their primary unit. The connection is very strong but the "family" only carried through birth lines. Neither concept is totally correct; there are DNA lines that flow through the families; however, there is a much stronger connection through the energetic field that held the world intact, connected, billions of years ago. The result of the initial explosion was a simple web. Today, the web is much more complex but it is still connected.

So why do we care? What difference does it make if we are energetically connected or not? It is very important if you understand that what I do affects you and what you do affects me even if I am in the United States and you are in Russia. What's more, it does not even have to be an action; it can be a thought that impacts us both, as Braden illustrated in a cross continental experiment. Therefore, we must be concerned because if one person is angry and hateful, that anger and hate will overflow to others. Maybe that person will lash out and take innocent lives, like the angry young man who gunned down 20 children and six staff members at Sandy Hook Elementary School in Newtown, Connecticut, on December 14, 2012. On the other hand, it may be more subtle, that one feels uncomfortable being around an angry person because of a sense that "something is just not quite right."

With all the anger, hate, killing, torture, rape, and general hostilities taking place in the world today, on every continent, in every country, in every town, you might say that you are not a part of it and it does not directly affect you, but it does. You are just not aware of it. This is a concrete case for the often-repeated phrase "Be the change you want to see in others."

What is that change we want to see in the world? Reduction of hostilities, hate, war, mean people, pain, road rage, suffering on both a personal and global scale is a good start. With what do we want to replace it? The Dalai Lama XIV once said, "Only the development of compassion and understanding for others can bring us the tranquility and happiness we all seek." If we can control our anger, fear, prejudice, and sense of separation, then as a result of mirroring (others will mimic what they see), the improvement will spread throughout the world. Change begins with each of us.

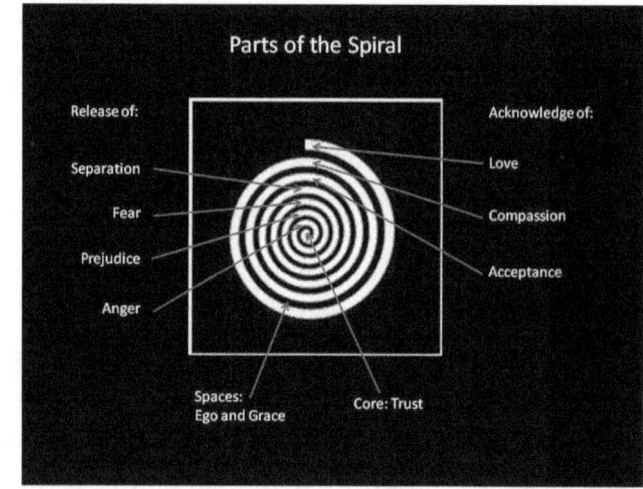

The spiral is used as the symbol for universal love, where *"love" is defined as the energy of the universe.* In the "Universal Spiral of Love," each layer of the spiral has its own meaning. It is in the meaning of the layers and in the spaces between the layers, that release of suffering and enlightenment is found.

Part One: Philosophy

Four Basic States of Human Ego Emotions

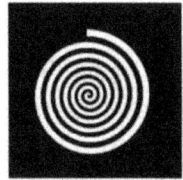

The first four layers of the spiral relate to ego traits of the natural human condition: anger, fear, prejudice, and separation are all behaviors that cause us pain and suffering. They also cause pain and suffering to others who interact with us when we are acting out any of the four traits. Our goal is to release these four ego traits from our consciousness and cellular being.

1 Release of Anger

The first layer of the spiral is "release of anger." Let's look at anger from a different perspective from what we normally consider. Shakyamuni Buddha said, "Anger is like a hot coal, it burns the hand of the one who holds it." Anger is used as an "emotion" or a "tool." If it is used as an emotion, the result of the anger is detrimental to the person using or holding it. It causes stress, raises blood pressure, and sets off various chemical processes in the body that are harmful to the organism. If anger is a tool, used in a conscious way rather than as an emotional response, it becomes a force that can be manipulative and damaging to others. Anger used as a tool often incorporates an element of intimidation to be effective. It may be used successfully to obtain a desired end result, but it comes at a high price to both the user and receiver.

Susan Forward, in her book *Toxic Parents: Overcoming Their Hurtful Legacy and Reclaiming Your Life,* quoted a victim of an angry parent who said:

> If I had to choose between physical and verbal abuse, I'd take a beating anytime. You can see the marks, so at least people feel sorry for you. With the verbal stuff, it just makes you crazy. The wounds are invisible. Nobody cares. Real bruises heal a hell of a lot faster than insults. (Forward 92)

Forward explains the long-term impact of cruel words and actions:

> When you take these negative opinions out of other people's mouths and put them into your unconscious, you are "internalizing" them. Internalization of negative opinions—changing "you are" to "I am"—forms the foundation of low self-esteem. Besides significantly impairing your sense of yourself as a lovable competent person, verbal abuse can create self-fulfilling negative expectations about how you will get along in the world. (Forward 110)

Part One: Philosophy

Anger as an emotion harms the body—anger as a tool harms the spirit. It changes the heart. Each time anger is used to obtain a specific end, the user's heart hardens a bit and sets in motion an addictive craving for the ego high that results: the sense of power, the absolute confidence of correctness, and a false sense of self-esteem. Our egos thrive on these inputs, but at the expense of using our hearts as fuel that is ultimately consumed.

In Les Carter's book, *The Anger Trap: Free Yourself from the Frustrations that Sabotage Your Life*, he describes the use of anger as a way to control others. If an angry person has complete control over the situation, actions, and thoughts of others, then those others might not be able to see the angry person's potential for being wrong. Such a person might believe that to be correct is to be loved and the best way to be correct is to coerce others through domination by anger. Carter also explains the importance of "freedom." This refers to the freedom everyone has to choose for themselves what to believe and do. He offers the following guidelines for understanding our personal freedom:

- All expressions of anger are the result of choices, not just unavoidable reactions.

- You can choose to drop coercion or manipulative efforts; your aim need not be to dominate or win.

- You can choose to address needs, preferences, and perceptions with a firm yet calm "disposition. You can choose to forgive or let go of your anger, not because you are supposed to do so, but because it makes sense. (Carter 70)

Carter concluded that "Recognizing it is delusional to think you can control the reactions and perceptions of others, you can discover a sense of liberation never known before" (71).

This is not to say that anger should never be used. In the case of a victim in the hands of an abuser, the victim often squelches and internalizes the anger that, in turn, causes severe damage to the soul and body. Instead, if the anger had been let out and directed at the abuser at the very first incident, further abuse might have been avoided. If that opportunity is missed, then anger becomes self-consuming for the victim.

We might say that sometimes anger is the only tool that will be effective to produce the desired results. This is not true. The recipient of the force has his or her own ego that feels under attack. On the surface, it may seem as though the recipient is complying, but in reality, he or she may institute some form of passive sabotage into the situation that is typically unseen by the inflictor at the time of the outburst or at a later date.

Karmic debt is accumulated on both people involved in the argument and they remain tied to each other in a damaging way if one of them does not release the anger chain. It is much more effective and without negative karmic debit to use compassionate wisdom and understanding to produce the desired effect instead of rage. The receiver of this intent is more likely to respond from the heart with sympathy and empathy to the situation. They are much more likely to make an honest attempt to resolve the issue in a creative and thoughtful manner.

Anger cuts off the creative energy of both people involved. It paralyzes them and inhibits the production of an effective resolution. Conversely, compassionate wisdom triggers our innate desire to be helpful problem solvers. The other person obtains a glowing sense of pride and ownership in working to resolve the situation.

2 Release of Fear

The second layer of the spiral is "release of fear."

There are two kinds of souls in this world—those that love to witness a robust electrical storm, Mother Nature celebrating with her own fireworks, and those that fear Mother Nature's stormy temper tantrums. Both types of souls witness exactly the same event, but interpret it quite differently.

Fear comes from not knowing the end result of an event. The mind of a fearful soul writes its own ending to a scenario instead of waiting for the scenario to be played out. The fearful soul might say "A bolt of lightning will strike me; the rising water in the streets will flood my home; the wind will blow the roof off my house." All are fears of the unknown.

Maybe in the past you lived through a terrible hurricane or tornado and witnessed firsthand damage like this occurring so you have a rational basis for your fear. If this is not the case, then your fears are nothing more than misplaced expectations. Feeling as though you have no control and are at the mercy of your circumstances creates fear.

For people who are plagued with panic and anxiety attacks, the fear arises from an irrational state of being that quite literally paralyzes them, preventing them from acting or thinking rationally. To change this reaction, they have to change the scenario playing out in their minds. Fear can be eradicated by simply changing how you view things and by relinquishing the need to control everything and everyone in the environment.

Change is inevitable. Absolutely nothing stays the same; therefore there is no need to become attached to any idea or thing. Once you replace your need to control the minutia of everyday life with the attitude that results from understanding that all things will change, your blood pressure will drop along with your heart rate. Your stress and fear will vanish. It is that simple.

Roger Walsh addresses fear in *Essential Spirituality: The Seven Central Practices to Awaken Heart and Mind.* He says: "Fear thrives in darkness and ignorance, but when we turn the light of awareness on it, it shrivels and transforms" (84). It's much easier and more comfortable to ignore our fears and deal with them only when we must. Walsh believes that to eliminate fear, we must thoroughly examine it from all aspects and run it through a reality check (88).

3 Release of Prejudice

The third layer of the spiral is "release of prejudice." Gordon Allport in *The Nature of Prejudice* offers an historical review of the word "prejudice" and with it numerous definitions of the word. The definition he seems to favor is "A feeling, favorable or unfavorable, toward a person or thing, prior to, or not based on, actual experience" (Allport 6). He says:

> There is a natural basis for this tendency. Life is so short, and the demands upon us for practical adjustments so great, that we cannot let our ignorance detain us in our daily transactions. We have to decide whether objects are good or bad by classes. We cannot weigh each object in the world by itself....*Prejudgments become prejudices only if they are not reversible when exposed to new knowledge.* [Emphasis his] (Allport 9)

Prejudice is an odd word. When we hear it, we typically think it means to have a dislike for someone of another race or religion. Alternatively, it may mean that we have a preference for one thing over another. However, if you break the word down into its parts to "pre" and "judge" it takes on a different meaning.

We pre-judge a situation when we make a decision without all of the facts; we jump to conclusions. In a sense, we are making up the scenario in our heads instead of letting it play out. It is our own story instead of reality. If we are pre-judging a person, we are making up stories about that person, laying our own colors and textures on him or her, not seeing that person for whom they really are. It is impossible for any one person to know the details of every situation or the thoughts and actions of another person. Because of this, our minds just fill in the blanks where there are holes in our knowledge.

In an example scenario, I am walking down a deserted street; I am alone. Ahead I see two young men on the other side of the street and they see me. They cross over to my side of the street, just ahead of me. My mind immediately tells me "I am about to be mugged!" My heart begins to pound faster, my blood pressure soars, and fear takes over my body and mind. As they get closer, they begin to speak: "Hey lady, stop a minute..." (absolute terror now) "... you dropped something back there, let me run and get it for you." One of the young men quickly retrieves my purse and hands it back to me and says, "Have a great day, ma'am." Then they walk on.

If you were in this situation, how would you feel after the young men leave? You might feel relief, embarrassment, or still clinging to the fear of what might have happened? Most likely gratitude is not what you are feeling because the intense fear resulting from your pre-judgment of the situation will not let you feel relief yet, but that is exactly what you should be feeling.

Every day, we pre-judge events and people in our lives. Every day we are wrong about the details but this does not stop us from continuing to do it. We are like gamblers; every once in a great while when we get it right, we win, so it reinforces our false beliefs that what we think is true.

Why do we create such stress in our lives? The answer is our ego's need to control everything, everyone, and every situation around us. We do not like surprises. We do not like the unknown. It is the fear of not knowing that causes us stress. Rationally, we know that everything changes in life but we cannot accept that for ourselves. Constant change for others is okay but we do not want it—leave me alone!

We need to let our own lives play out without assumptions and pre-judgments of others and events. Stay in the moment, mindful of what is actually happening instead of what you think is or will be happening. Relax. Have fun with life and stop trying to guess the next act in this play called life. We just need to laugh at the scene we are in at this precise moment. Laughter is the best medicine for heart disease and curing prejudice.

Don Miquel Ruiz says in his book *The Four Agreements:*

> We have the tendency to make assumptions about everything. The problem with making assumptions is that we *believe* they are the truth…We make assumptions about what others are doing or thinking—we take it personally—then we blame them and react by sending emotional poison with our word….All the sadness and drama you have lived in your life was rooted in making assumptions and taking things personally. The whole world of control between humans is about making assumptions and taking things personally. (Ruiz 63-64)

Kosho Niwano also addresses the issue of making assumptions in *The Buddha in Everyone's Heart: Seeking the World of the Lotus Sutra*:

> We are the ones who create the difficulty, by thinking "This is how things ought to be" rather than recognizing things as they actually are. Difficulties arise when we try to "solve" problems. We judge certain phenomena to be antagonistic and hard to deal with and thus create troublesome problems for ourselves. We should concentrate on perceiving the Buddha-nature in people and viewing them with warmth and an attitude of Buddhist compassion. That is the great path. (Niwano 169)

Part One: Philosophy

4 Release of Separation

The fourth layer of the spiral is "release of separation." This layer concerns the fallacy of the idea that we are all independent people and refers to being separated from others because of this "independence."

The term "separation" could have a negative connotation with its usual definition—to depart from; to break into parts; to divide a whole into pieces and move the pieces apart. When it comes to relationships, separation can be painful, such as in the breakup of a marriage or a child leaving the family nest. Separation comes at the price of loneliness and pain. Even when we want out of a relationship, in the period immediately after the separation, we experience a feeling of loss.

Can we really completely separate from those with whom we have had a connection? No, we may physically move away; however, there is a residue that will always be there forever, connecting the two energetically. From the aspect of physics, humans are energetic beings; we are forever connected to each and every other person or energetic being on the planet. Taking it to the next level, we are connected energetically to everything on the planet and in fact in the universe.

We are all part of the whole of existence—a link that can never be severed—not even by the physical death of our material bodies. We are part of the whole; we always have been, are currently, and will always be part of the whole. What each of us thinks and does, sends a ripple effect out into the universe and affects it all.

Consider, how it is possible for two people to walk into a room; one lights up the room, the other saps it of energy. How is it possible for these two opposite scenarios to be real? Why is it that we are inexplicably drawn or repelled by the energy of others? This is because we are energetically connected to the universe, everything, and everyone in it. A classic example of how we can be impacted by a single element—water—illustrates this point. Without water all life as we know it on this planet would die. If all the water on the planet dried up and it never rained, snowed, or became humid with fog or mist ever again, physical life would die.

It's important for us to understand our inseparable connection with the universe. Our despair, our loneliness, our sense of rejection, being left out, is all just a façade, our physical minds playing a trick! Not only is it impossible to separate ourselves, but we are all exactly the same! We are all part of the same whole. Therefore, if we are all part of the same whole, how can we be anything but equal? There is no hierarchy, no being "less than," no being superior or inferior, no lacking—just "is."

Fear causes us to place judgment on others because we are fearful of the connection. We are fearful of the full potential of what that connection might mean for us as an "individual," which in and of itself is a myth. Therefore, if we let go of the fear of separation and accept that you, I, and the rest of humanity, are one, then the only name we need to call others is "love." It is impossible for relationships to be anything but positive if we all recognize the truth of our existence. We are all the same, connected, identical, a branch of a branch called "love."

The question becomes, why do we feel so disconnected and separate from others? Many theorists believe that it is based our individual egos. Tarthang Tulku in *Reflections of the Mind: Western Psychology Meets Tibetan Buddhism* talks about what happens when we buy into the image that is formed by our ego. He says that when we develop our self-image, the ego immediately begins to take over. The more we are convinced that the image that we create is really who we are, the more problems we create for ourselves. "The more rigid and proud the ego, the greater the awareness of its own fragility. There is a fear of loss of identity or loss of objects and persons whom we unconsciously include as part of our identity" (Tulku113). The ego convinces us that if we lose this identity, then chaos will ensue and we will lose control. As a result, the ego goes on the defensive to protect this carefully crafted image. Tulku says "Denial, repression, rationalization, escape, compromise, camouflage, rigid character traits, and other mechanisms all function further to complicate the samsaric [hellish]situation" (Tulku113).

If we internalize and accept the fourth layer of the spiral, release of separation, then we realize that we are all one; we have all that we could ever need; we are whole, and that all of this pain can be avoided.

How do we know when we are acting from our ego—the false self or our true self? In Deepak Chopra's book, *Twenty Spiritual Lessons for Creating the Life You Want: The Way of the Wizard*, he answers this question. The book is the story of how the wizard Merlin prepares young Arthur to be a successful ruler. In a conversation about why Merlin lives backwards, he grows young instead of old, Merlin states that we humans are nothing but energy. Of course, Arthur is bewildered:

> Because you identify with this body, you think you need a form. Energy is formless, so you think it cannot be you. But, I was only pointing out that energy can't be born; it has no beginning or end. Until you stop thinking of yourself as having a beginning, you'll never find the deathless part of yourself, which must be unborn if it is never to die (Chopra 44).

Merlin also tried to teach Arthur that he is not the role that he plays, a boy, son of his parents, someone who likes to talk to animals, et cetera; nor is he the thoughts that form in his mind. It is when we are not thinking and not playing our roles, when we simply respond to the beauty of our world, when we first awaken in the morning and our mind is clear for that split second before we begin the chatter of the day that is being who we are, not the role we are playing (Chopra 39).

Part One: Philosophy

Three Higher States of Spiritual Essences

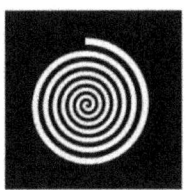

As we have seen, anger, fear, prejudice, and separation are all behaviors that cause us and others who interact with us pain and suffering. Our goal is to release them from our consciousness, and cellular being. The next three layers of the spiral are symbolic of traits that lie at the core of our spiritual essence. These traits counter balance our human baggage: acceptance, compassion, and love are our connection to the universe. With the three spiritual traits, our goal is to recognize, acknowledge, and fully believe that we are one with the energy of acceptance, compassion, and love; these traits are innate within us though we typically do not recognize them.

5 Acknowledging Acceptance

The first spiritual trait is "acceptance." In some quarters, the mere idea of acceptance of any idea other than our own is a cause for conflict. In U.S. politics, neither side will accept anything the other side does, even if they themselves once proposed it when they were in power. In religion, where one faith claims to be the one true "God-chosen" group, of course, no one of differing faiths would ever accept that concept or they would just change faiths to become a "chosen one."

Many people, including top scientists, buy into the phrase "Don't believe it unless you see it." To accept that something is true without irrefutable confirmed evidence is difficult for some people. Why is this? What purpose does this rigid stance serve? Does it really matter if one cannot prove absolutely an idea before we buy into it?

What we believe does matter because we only act according to what we believe. Therefore, if we believe we are the only "God-chosen" people on the face of the planet then our attitude and behavior towards others will reflect superiority and be uncompromising. If we believe ourselves to be unworthy of living a happy life, then we will live an unhappy life. If we believe that we must fight for what is justly ours, always fighting for our piece of the pie, then we will always have a sense of lacking and we will spend our whole lives like Don Quixote, tilting at windmills. If we are raised to believe that through hard work, dedication, focus, with a bit of luck mixed in, we can accomplish anything, then that is exactly what we will do.

Part One: Philosophy

The human mind is capable of creating its own reality; what it thinks is what it creates. It is unlikely that anyone consciously says to himself, "I want a hard life." Even those who become successful suicide bombers believe they are doing it for their faith and believe their actions will be richly rewarded. Therefore, if we want to live a happier, easier life, why not stop believing we have to fight for everything. We need to stop believing the world is out to get us. Stop believing our lives must be full of obstacles that we must struggle to overcome. There is no reason to create these realities for ourselves when it is unnecessary.

Tara Brach, in *Radical Acceptance: Embracing Your Life with the Heart of a Buddha*, illustrated this concept of letting go of our struggle and just being calm with ourselves in the moment. She told the story of Jacob, a man who was in the middle stages of Alzheimer's disease. He was aware of his deteriorating faculties. He had moments of both lucidity and confusion. One day he was teaching Buddhism to a class of meditation students. Once in front of the room, he completely forgot why he was there.

> Putting his palms together at his heart, Jacob started naming aloud what was happening: "Afraid embarrassed, confused, feeling like I'm failing, powerless, shaking, sense of dying, sinking, lost." For several more minutes he sat, head slightly bowed, continuing to name his experience. As his body began to relax and his mind grew calmer, he also noted that aloud. At last Jacob lifted his head, looked slowly around at those gathered and apologized. Many of the students were in tears. As one put it, "No one has ever taught us like this. Your presence has been the deepest teaching." ... In some fundamental way, he didn't create an adversary out of feelings of fear and confusion. He didn't make anything wrong... Nothing is wrong—whatever is happening is just "real life." (Brach 74)

If we buy into the concept that all things are just as they should be at that moment in time then things change. We should accept that events take place around us to give us an opportunity to grow and learn. Accept that there is *always* more than one way to believe and act and that is all right for it to be so. Accept that there is no separation among us and we are all part of the same whole. If we can accept these as truths, then we will stop fighting with ourselves.

Deepak Chopra, in *The Seven Spiritual Laws of Success*, discusses "acceptance" in terms of his Fourth Law—The Law of Least Effort. Generally, this law states that if you do less you will accomplish more. The first component of this law is acceptance.

> Acceptance simply means that you make a commitment. "Today, I will accept people, situations, circumstances, and events as they occur." This means I will know that this moment is as it should be, because the whole universe is as it should be. This moment—the one you're experiencing right now—is the culmination of all the moments you have experienced in the past. This moment is as it is because the entire

universe is as it is. When you struggle against this moment, you're actually struggling against the entire universe. (Chopra 57)

When we accept that your reality is right and necessary for you; my reality is right and necessary for me; and the world will not come to an end because of the existences of [seemingly] separate realities; then we can let go of rigid thinking that leads to suffering.

If we accept that the philosophy of cause and effect is true, then we understand everything that happens to us is directly related to some condition that we ourselves put into play. We then put ourselves in the driver's seat to change our own destiny. By taking full responsibility for our own lives then we can change what we do not want. When we change our attitude, we change our life.

A man who has a few dollars in his pocket may consider himself to be lacking, not having enough and therefore be sad. Alternatively, he can believe himself to be fortunate to have those few dollars and be happy. His reality, his state of being can change, when he changes his attitude. If you want a happy stress-free life, then stop hanging on to the idea that you are unhappy and stressed out. Accept that you are in a learning situation, learn what you need to learn and move on.

Absolutely nothing is exactly the same as it was just a second ago. If you believe your life is dull and unchanging that is only in your head. You have blinders on and are not seeing the truth—your truth. Life changes—things change—you change.

Nikkyo Niwano, in *Buddhism for Everyday Life,* tells us, "Since all things are constantly changing, clinging to the past only causes suffering. At the same time, troubles can lead to improvements. Bitter failures, in other words, can become the building blocks for future success (Niwano 34).

We must recognize that we play a role in creating our own pain and do something else. The old adage that "Insanity is doing the same thing over and over but expecting different results" is true. If we want a different life, we must accept that we alone have the control sticks to change our situation. Cause and effect, we are the "cause" that "effects" our reality and only we can create the reality we want.

6 Acknowledging Compassion

The second spiritual trait is "compassion."Compassion—real compassion—is different from fatherly, benevolent compassion. Real compassion does not look down upon others, feel sorry for them, and therefore want to help. This response is not helpful, it carries overtones of judgment. The Dalai Lama XIV, in *The Art of Happiness,* said:

> Compassion can be roughly defined in terms of a state of mind that is non-violent, non-harming, and non-aggressive. It is a mental attitude based on the wish for others to be free of their suffering and is associated with a sense of commitment, responsibility, and respect towards others. (Lama 114)

He explains that there are two types of compassion. The first is the normal, ordinary type that "is tinged with attachment"—the feeling of controlling someone, or loving someone so that person will love you back. When the object of your compassion does something you do not like, that compassion can easily turn to hatred because of the attachment. Genuine compassion, he says, is different.

> Genuine compassion is based on the rationale that all human beings have an innate desire to be happy and overcome suffering, just like myself. And, just like me, they have the natural right to fulfill this fundamental aspiration. On the basis of the recognition of this equality and commonality, you develop a sense of affinity and closeness with others. With this as a foundation, you can feel compassion regardless of whether you view the other person as a friend or an enemy. It is based on the other's fundamental rights rather than your own mental projection. Upon this basis, then, you will generate love and compassion. That's genuine compassion. (Lama 115)

Compassion is judgment-free. It is clean and sparkling, warm and loving. It is supportive yet not carrying the weight of others—others need to carry their own weight to heal themselves. Compassion is listening, it is being there at the right time, and the right place to be a sounding board, a shoulder to lean on without engaging your mouth. Compassion can only be felt; it is not an action, it is a state of being; it is a radiance that engulfs others in a cloud of warmth and security. There is a feeling of expansiveness, of being energized and calm at the same time. There is a sense of the heart being the center of all that is.

You cannot extend compassion to others if you do not have it within yourself to extend. However, the Dalai Lama believes that it is within all of us; it just may not be activated. You must take time out of your daily routine to service the needs of the physical body to activate compassion in the spiritual essence. Compassion is not a characteristic of the physical; it comes from our core essence and permeates out to the physical.

If compassion were part of the physical, only skin deep, then it would be ego, condescension-filled support for the benefit of ourselves instead of the one who is suffering. That is the nature of the physical self—it cannot help it. The physical self is charged with providing the protective shell for us while in body. Consequently, it will naturally put you first. However, when the spiritual self has activated compassion, it overwhelms the ego of the physical mind and radiates out, extending to any pain it encounters. It does not fix the pain of others, it only calms their physical body and mind enough so that their own spiritual care can be activated, felt, and heard.

The question becomes then, how should we extend compassion to others? Our conversations and comments to others should be filled with understanding and compassion. For our part, we should mostly listen; listen for the pain and suffering of others to pour out. Without telling them what to do, we should gently guide their thinking toward considering the root of their pain. They must discover the reasons on their own to have the desire and strength to make the corrections. We should however, talk generally about the primary causes of suffering: incorrectly making all events around us about ourselves, attachment issues, forgetting who we really are, and thinking we are alone in this world.

The tools to end suffering are simple to use. Simplicity is the key to understanding. Compassion is the cement to secure the truths into their physical beings.

George Mullins, in *Raising Up Bodhisattvas in the Modern Ages,* discusses the importance of compassion. He said, "Unless one works unselfishly and untiringly for the salvation of others, he has no salvation himself. Individual salvation alone is not true salvation." He indicates that in Buddhism, compassion is much more than simply a kind act; it involves seeing the Buddha-nature (inherent ability to become an enlightened buddha) in everyone.

> Reaching out to people in their suffering, whether or not that suffering is apparent to them, is a means to acquaint them to this truth for no other reason than to develop the Buddha potential within them joyfully. Without recognizing the oneness of all people and acting appropriately, people cannot be who they ought to be—buddha(s). This is compassion. (Mullins 90)

Nikkyo Niwano, in *Buddhism for Everyday Life,* echoes this theme. He wrote:

> Compassion is at once the wish to make others happy and the desire to take away their pain and suffering....We can demonstrate our compassion by helping others not only to unburden themselves of their pain and suffering but also to cleanse their souls so that they can find new ways to live meaningful and happy lives. This is the ultimate expression of compassion, the ultimate act of bodhisattva caring. (Niwano 167-168)

7 Acknowledging Love

The third spiritual trait and the last of the seven layers of the spiral is "love." Love is not last because it is of least importance. It is last because it wraps all the other layers in love and sends it out into the universe. Love is frequently called by other names: universal life force energy (or just universal energy), God, Buddha, Allah, spirit, source, and the light. Love energy is different from the energy of compassion—you need both. Love is the force that keeps our physical protective shell alive. When the shell can no longer function, the love energy simply moves on to a different plane to reflect and prepare for reentry into a different protective shell.

Love is all that is. Love is the glue that holds everything in existence together. Love is non-judgmental. Love is non-prejudicial—it does not shower on one more favorable than on another—it just is. How can "God" shine his light more favorably on any one group of people when all people are made of the exact same substance—an energy called God is just another name for love.

There are far too many people in the world today who dislike themselves, have low self-esteem, and consider themselves unworthy. It is the ego at play, the physical shell trying to steal the show, so to speak. The body wants to be center stage, not unlike a two-year old child. When children want attention, they do not distinguish between good and bad attention, to them it is all the same. So it is, with the ego mind of the physical body. It creates these ideas of being less than or unworthy, just to get attention and we do feed it. We keep this fallacy, this myth alive because the body wants to focus on itself instead of its core essence—you as who you are—love.

Since we are taught from birth that everything is either good or bad, it is hard to imagine an existence without judgment. It is bad to cry all night long and good to sleep, bad to touch the stove, good to play nicely with others, bad to hit others, good to hug others, bad to cheat, but good to study hard, and so on. Yet that is exactly what love is, existence without judgment. Love just is.

Love carries with it or is composed of all of the knowledge of the universe (and beyond) of the past, present, and future. Nothing just disappears. No action just ceases. The consequences of it ripple throughout the energy field and remain, as a record of events. It is not stored with a label of good or bad—it is just an event, with its consequences duly noted. This is why any act of kindness is so important. No act is too small; they all have ripple effects that can be felt far and wide for an eternity.

Deepak Chopra, in *Twenty Lessons for Creating the Life You Want*, defines love in a very similar fashion:

> There is a force of love present everywhere, it can be trusted to bring your own life into order and peace....No thread has been dropped in that immense time span; every piece of information and energy has evolved in such a way to make it possible for you, the observer, to look into a cosmos that is the living picture of your entire past...Things could have taken very different directions, in fact an infinity of directions, that would not have resulted in what you recognize as yourself. What allows this balancing act to take place is organization and intelligence. As the wizard sees it, order cannot simply spring from randomness; it is innate in creation. Thus, the titanic forces swirling through the cosmos do not war with one another; they are

allowed to exist and evolve as part of nature's tendency toward growth. Now take all these qualities together: order, balance, evolution, and intelligence. What you have is a description of love. It is not the popular ideal, it is the wizard's love—the force that upholds life and nurtures it. (Chopra 62)

How do we use this thing called love? We do not have to "use" it. It is there for us to tap into whenever we need a solution, or uplifting, whenever our physical protector shell needs grounding in reality. We need only to remember who and what we really are—love.

We should accept that we are pure. Accept that everyone has access to all the knowledge available. Accept that we are not bad or good, better than or less than, everyone is all the same—equal. Somehow, we just need to silence the ego mind fighting for attention. When we consciously try to keep judgment out of our life—out of our ego mind, then we are able to experience our true and natural being—love.

Part One: Philosophy

Part One: Philosophy

Between the Lines and the Core of the Spiral

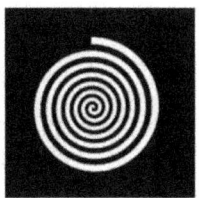

Naturally in a spiral, there are spaces between the lines and a core to provide support and motivation.

8 Between the Layers—Ego and Grace

The inner lines or layers of the spiral that relate to the physical body are entirely bound by ego. The ego lies in the spaces between the lines of the spiral. As you move to the three spiritual traits, the ego in the spaces morphs into universal energy-consciousnesses, mindful, spiritual purposeful energy. It can also be call grace. It saturates and supports the actions of acceptance and compassion. Without the spaces on both sides of the lines to support it, the behaviors would collapse back down into the four human traits.

This idea can also be interpreted that the four human traits, without ego to support them, would open up into grace or the universal energy called love. The last line of the spiral or last layer (love or the actual energy of the universe) is just symbolic. It does not need to be present for those who have totally incorporated the thoughts, intentions, and actions of acceptance and compassion. For most people who are floating among the layers, it helps to keep the universal energy of love tightly compacted around them to give them the extra support they need—we need—as humans.

Therefore, there are two bodies, the four inner qualities that represent the physical and the three outer qualities that represent the spiritual or energetically connected self. Both have their boundary influences but they are interlocked as one. It is a continuous line spiral, not a series of nested unconnected boxes where the flow from one thought, intention, and/or action is disjointed. The spiral shows the fluidity of transformation, ease of backsliding, or ease of moving forward with the appropriate support.

9 Core of the Spiral—Trust

Trust must be at the center of the spiral. When you release the inner four levels, you trust that, in fact, they are being released. Remember that although you may release them one minute, if you choose to respond to situations with anger, fear, prejudice, or separation, then you are inviting them back in.

The way the human mind works is that our mouth can be saying one thing but our mind and heart believe the opposite or we might believe what we are saying is just wishful thinking, a prayer for it to happen. As long as this is the case then the release does not really happen. There is a loosening a bit of the ropes but bondage remains.

"Bondage" is a good word for what happens when we believe we cannot really change because we tie ourselves to our previous mistakes and repeat them. It is only through trust, real trust, in ourselves and our ability to control our destiny that we will actually be able to change course.

Trust is like believing in magic, ghosts, or miracles. If one truly believes in magic, magic happens. It may not be the sudden appearance of a Lamborghini with a clear title bearing your name, but something magical will occur on a transformational level if you are open to seeing it. Thus, it is with releasing anger, fear, prejudice, and separation from your life. Old habits are just that and habits can be changed. Change happens only if you believe you are behind the control panel of your life, you are the "wizard behind the curtain."

Once we accept and trust that everything is placed in our path for a reason then life becomes much easier to live. We no longer second-guess events; we just go with the flow. This works because every decision we make is also the right decision for that exact moment. If the results of that decision seem to be "disastrous," they really are not, it is just another opportunity to learn. If the results are "positive," then we also will have the opportunity to learn from that too.

This works best when we trust in the process. The events do not change because you trust or not trust; the events will happen based upon cause and effect. If you trust that you can influence those events with your attitude and beliefs then it all flows easier. Life is easier.

We started out talking about trusting our ability to change and control our lives then we moved to trusting the universe to present what is best for us based on cause and effect. We now come back to trusting our ability to work with and learn from the universe. This seems circular, however it is not really a circle, it is more like the spiral. This is because each time we learn, we make changes, and when we go with the flow, we grow and expand outward, just like the spiral.

So while we call the spiral the symbol of universal love, it in itself is also the symbol for personal and universal trust. There is no need to add anything to the symbology of the spiral to indicate trust; it is already there. Love, acceptance, compassion, and trust—what more do you need for a successful life? Nothing.

Part One: Philosophy

10 Spirals as Symbols

Throughout time man has used symbols to project meaning. The earliest forms of writing are petrography and cuneiforms, which are both picture-based writing systems. Each picture represents a thing or action.

What does a spiral mean? It has been used by many cultures over time as a strong foundational symbol; each culture interprets it in its own way. Spiritually or energetically the spiral means "all encompassing forever." In life, we start out with little knowledge. In our first lifetime and the beginning of each lifetime as we grow and develop, we are presented with scenarios to learn the same basic principles: how to alleviate or detach from anger, fear, prejudice, and separation and instead realize that we are acceptance, compassion, and love. Over and over we find ourselves presented with learning opportunities and each time we learn just a bit more. The spiral reflects not only the repetition of learning but growth after each trial, moving outwards.

Growth Spiral

1. Begin with your base knowledge and problems
2. Gradually gain momentum for understanding, comfortably and easily
3. Help others
4. Personal struggle and need help to push through it.
5. Period of rest
7. Begin again

Spirals also reflect the all-encompassing nature of love—the outer layer of the spiral. It is a protective shell that permits us the opportunity to learn at whatever pace we require. It permeates all that we do with the universal knowledge of all time so that the answers we seek are always available to use, in the form that we can hear and understand for our level of development at that moment in time.

The spiral also represents the foundational behavior for learning and growth that is giving and taking. We give of ourselves to help others in their times of need to detach from their sources of suffering, and we accept help from others when we are mired in our own muck and cannot find a way out.

Oddly, it is the acceptance of help from others that seems to be more problematic for people than giving help. This is why the first and foremost practice of life is to help others. When we do, we learn something about ourselves in the process. It also conditions us to be sympathetic and empathetic to life's painful events, which every one of us will experience at some point in every lifetime. So when those same events happen to us, we recognize that we will end the pain faster by asking for help.

If we never ask for help, we will continue to stew much longer than is necessary. We will eventually figure it out enough to rise from the muck, but with help, it is always less painful. By requesting help, we give others the opportunity to give help. So our fates are interwoven in the fabric of life.

11 How to Use the Spiral for Personal Growth and Healing

You can obtain many beneficial results from implementing the practical exercises in this book. Your mental health will improve. Your relationships with family, friends, and co-workers will improve. And last but certainly not least, your physical health will improve. Working through the exercises will take time; absolutely you cannot complete them all in just one week. What you can and should do is to start with implementing this first practice on a daily basis. It is recommended that you read aloud this verse the first thing upon awakening and the last thing before retiring at night.

This exercise will begin the change you desire on an energetic level first, which eventually will begin to work on a cellular level. Once your physical body begins to shift, your behaviors and thought patterns will change too. At this point, you will certainly begin to feel a release of suffering and gain a deep sense of peace and gratitude.

Part One: Philosophy

When you read the verse, the purity of intent is the most important aspect to allow the energy to work. Begin by saying:

> **I am part of the light;**
> **I am the love of the universe.**
> **All sentient beings are part of the same divine loving energy.**
> **I will live, believe and act as one.**
> **Whatever I think and do will have a ripple effect into the universe.**
> **If I project pain and anger, so it will be.**
> **If I project acceptance and love of all that is, so it will be.**
> **Whenever my thoughts and actions reflect this, healing will occur.**
> **Dis-ease will be released when there is no separation or distinction.**
> **All are one.**

With your fingers, draw the spiral in the palm of both hands, and then draw it over your heart. Begin drawing the spiral at the center, inner layer, and work outward. While doing this, say the following, one line for each layer of the spiral. It should be said at the conclusion of each layer drawn:

- **I release all my anger**
- **I release all my fear.**
- **I release all my prejudice.**
- **I release all my separation.**
- **I am acceptance.**
- **I am compassion.**
- **I am love.**

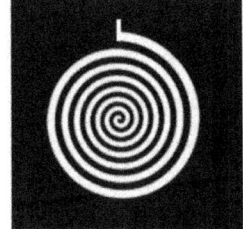

After the symbol is drawn over both palms and heart, say:

In all my thoughts and actions, I am one with all. I trust that all this is true.

Notice that the image of the healing spiral is slightly different from basic spiral. There is a line extended upward on the last layer. This is the extension of the love layer (universal energy, God, spiritual energy) out into the universe and strengthens your direct connection with the universe.

In the beginning, you probably will not believe that you are really able to release the four ego traits. Maybe you believe that you are not really acceptance, compassion, and love. However, with honest desire to improve and mindful behavioral changes, you will in fact be able to personify the traits and your true inner perfection will be revealed.

The practices in this book will not be easy, but they will be rewarding. This first practice is actually the easiest and at the same time it is extremely powerful. It is a good place to start.

12 Conclusion

When we live a life fully in the present, when we are mindful of each action, when our inner voices that cause us to suffer because of anger, fear, pre-judgment, and separation are silenced, then our lives become immeasurably easier. Human ego naturally draws us there but our repeated acquiescence establishes the habit that engrains sufferings within us.

When we accept that we are not alone in this world, that we are all energetically connected, that what I do does impact you and what you do does impact me, then we begin to treat others and ourselves with increased kindness and compassion.

When we consciously change our habits and live our lives based in acceptance of the learning gifts (challenges) given to us each day—gifts that we understand are in our highest good both spiritually and physically—then it is much easier to respond with compassion.

Compassion as a habit actually feels good. It is an addictive energy that the spiritual body, bound by the ego, craves. Once the habit of acceptance is established, the resulting compassion entices the physical body to develop a craving for the peace and serenity it brings. The ego will also eventually see that it is in its own interest to allow itself to be bathed in the loving healing energy. The ego is not stupid; it is just fearful. It wants to control what it does not understand. By establishing acceptance and compassion as habits, the ego now wants to exude control through these spiritual behaviors.

The establishment of acceptance and compassion can be considered a love habit. It has the effect of the physical body innately understanding and consciously becoming one with the spiritual body—the universal life force energy. We already are one with the spiritual body, but typically the ego, in its natural state does not recognize this. With the love habit, it does.

Once the love habit is established, the peace the physical mind obtains is strong enough virtually to eliminate backsliding. This makes complete sense—for once we experience what it is like to live without anger, fear, resentment, frustration, stress, and anxiety in our lives—once we live a life of peace, calm, and clearer thinking from a compassionate heart—who would want to go back? The spiritual body and the physical body become in tune, acting as one instead of as opposites. The turmoil of being pulled in two directions vanishes and we are firmly on a path of spiritual, physical contentment, and peace in this life.

The rest of the book provides short readings that will help you to understand better how to put these ideas into practice. Part Two directly relates to these specific attitude changes. Part Three introduces additional behavioral changes that support and enhance the foundational practices of the spiral. A good way to use the stories is to read, reflect, and complete the exercises one a day over a period of two months. If you only read the stories, roots of change will not be able to find firm grounding or nutrients. The exercises are intended to be introspective and provide the opportunity to make a real change in your life.

Part One: Philosophy

Part Two: Practices

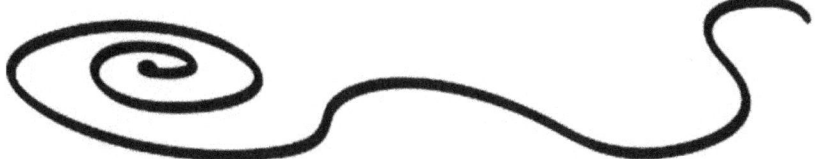

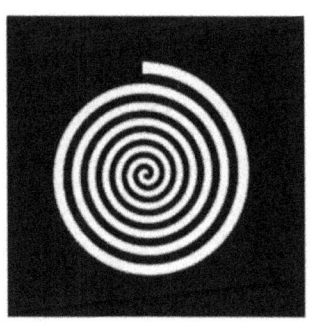

Part Two: Practices

Reflective Readings to Illustrate Each Layer of the Spiral

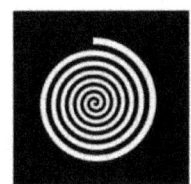

This section provides readings and exercises related to changing specific attitudes.

13 Release of Anger

Anger is the tightly wound inner layer. Anger and the next layer fear cause you to draw within yourself and try to shield yourself from the world. It is the most self-destructive of the four ego traits and behaviors that cause inner suffering. Anger is the strongest, most resilient, and unrelenting because we feel we have a right to our anger. We think the person with whom we are angry "did something to me, I have a right to be angry and I am NOT going to forgive!" In fact, there are more reasons to forgive than to hold onto the pain.

Picking Weeds

If you have ever tried to maintain a beautiful garden or yard you are well aware of the superfast growing nature of weeds. Even when there is a lack of rain for many weeks and everything else in nature has long since withered, weeds are growing strong. There are even weed trees and weed bushes that have been left to flourish while all else dies.

We can say that in the garden of our life, anger is our weeds. If we do not pluck them out, prevent them from growing at the moment they appear, anger will sprout its many extensions, dig its roots into our hearts, and suck the life out of any other positive emotion and attitude we have. Flowering happiness does not grow where there are acres of weeds. Blossoms of self-esteem are crowded out of the garden of life by clinging vines of anger. Compassion for our self and family is overcome by the prickly spines of weedy anger. Untempered anger destroys our lives just as surely as unattended weeds destroy the beauty of gardens.

It doesn't have to be like this because there are life tools just like there are garden tools. Anger like weeds must be removed at the root, not just mowed over. The best tool for removing anchor roots is forgiveness. Forgive others for whatever you think they did or did not do. Forgive yourself for what you believe you did or did not do or that you should have done.

Like weeds, anger never goes away on its own. It may lie dormant and appear to have been resolved but at the next transgression of self or others, it flares up and compounds the new issue.

Only forgiveness, true actual forgiveness, can remove the roots of anger. You will find that forgiveness has another powerful characteristic too. If you have truly forgiven someone, the next time an issue arises between you and that person, you will be much less likely to respond in anger. There is a residual effect of forgiveness that can last for the season of your life. How long the residual lasts depends on your ability to see things as they truly are without your own ego and emotional overlay.

So keep "forgiveness" and it sister tool "I am sorry" in your tool bag; hang them on your belt so you can have quick access to them at a moment's notice.

Your life's garden will stay in bloom for many seasons to come.

Exercise: Forgiveness—Part I

Write out your responses in the spaces provided.

Is there something that you feel guilty about having done to someone else? Write it down with as much detail as you can remember. Do not place blame on anyone else; own your own part. Be objective and state the facts of the situation without judgment.

How did the incident(s) make you feel at the time?

Part Two: Practices

How did the other person(s) involved feel at the time?

What could you have done or said differently that would have changed the situation?

Visualize having a conversation with that person(s). Write down the conversation between the two of you. If possible speak directly with the other person. Make amends for your part and forgive the other person.

Societal Anger

In addition to personal anger that we carry around with us, we also carry societal anger. This is an inherited set of emotional beliefs that can be handed down to us from our ancestral line or it can be adopted through our association with aspirational groups.

Aspirational groups consist of people for whom we aspire to be like. They can be a collection of individuals that all think the same way or actual organized groups that have formal ties or informational associations. For whatever reason, the group's stance makes sense and speaks to us; therefore, we adopt their views as our own.

What is interesting is that the higher level of emotion, the louder and angrier the tone, the more we listen. Subconsciously, we think "something they believe in that strongly must be important and true or they would not be so emotional about it."

Actually the opposite is true, when our beliefs are in line with the just and loving nature of the universe, we have no need to loudly defend them, they feel right to us and others. When those beliefs are prejudicial, unjust, stingy, or self-serving, then we need to shout them loud enough to convince ourselves and others they are true. There is a background white noise—it is the sound of compassion and love that emanates from the very earth upon which we walk. This also exists in the air that we breathe, a by-product of the universal force that connects all things and people that exist. We are bathed in this loving compassionate energy so if a message of exclusion, prejudice, favoritism, fear, or anger is to be heard, it must be shouted loudly. It must be emotionally charged to play to the prehistoric portion of our brain that has not evolved over the millennia of evolution, the amygdale. This is where fear and anger-based emotions are held and from where selfish ego-based decisions are made. Because the nature of our own physical bodies is to protect our essence—spiritual core, Buddha-nature, God within—the amygdale fires up to throw an angry shield around us. It tries to control all that it can, which includes the behavior and attitudes of others. It does not consider that what is good for me might not be good for you. It does not consider that there might be more than one truth. It believes that my truth is the only truth and if you do not accept my truth for yourself, then you are my enemy to be destroyed.

Since we live in a democracy, we use words instead of bullets (most of the time, thankfully!) to try to beat our enemies into submission. Our fear-based ego must dominate and so a war using words, hateful ones, are fired at the enemy who dares to believe differently. The firing of guns creates loud noises. The firing of words must also be loud to drown out the natural ambient sounds of love and compassion, the more false the message, the louder the firing must be, to be heard.

Stop firing. Change aspirational groups. Turn off the hate-mongering pundits on the airwaves. Read different printed words, words of acceptance, compassion, and love for all.

The latest figures say that two-thirds of Americans are overweight. Other studies show that Americans have the highest percentage of anxiety disorders in the world and our stress factors are also way beyond our global neighbors. It is well known that stress and anxiety cause people to eat more and exercise less.

The bombardment of selfish, fearful, angry, and controlling messages that play to our amygdale stress center in the brain is making us physically unhealthy. Since this is societal anger, it is prevalent where ever we go. We cannot escape it even if we don't buy into it; it still has a major impact on us.

We must find a way to be comfortable with diversity to lower our reflexive fear control response. We must find a way to turn down the volume of anger and fear so that the soothing atmospheric sounds of love and compassion can heal our hearts and souls. When we do this, the amygdale can relax, and let go of fear and let go of the need to control others. Let go of the anger it feels toward itself for being fearful and others for not obeying it. We can coexist with people who believe and act differently than we do. When everyone believes that diversity is acceptable and natural, then our sameness is revealed! Isn't that what we wanted in the first place – "them" to be like us?

Exercise: Forgiveness—Part II

Everyone has trigger points; when someone pushes our buttons, we become fearful or angry to cover our fear. What are your trigger points? How do you typically respond?

Part Two: Practices

Dig deep to uncover the real underlying reason for your fear.

```
┌─────────────────────────────────────────────────────────────┐
│                                                             │
│                                                             │
│                                                             │
│                                                             │
└─────────────────────────────────────────────────────────────┘
```

Is the fear real or imagined? Is the fear related to a situation that no longer exists? Examine your fear in terms of your current life situation, is there any connection to your current reality?

```
┌─────────────────────────────────────────────────────────────┐
│                                                             │
│                                                             │
│                                                             │
│                                                             │
└─────────────────────────────────────────────────────────────┘
```

How would your life change if you did let go of the fear? Would you be happier without the fear? If so, can you let go? If not, why not?

```
┌─────────────────────────────────────────────────────────────┐
│                                                             │
│                                                             │
│                                                             │
│                                                             │
└─────────────────────────────────────────────────────────────┘
```

Getting Even

"Don't get mad, get even." This concept has been around for centuries. Shakespeare used the theme in many of his tragedies. Unfortunately, this theme has also caused immeasurable number of wars and resulted in billions of deaths of people whose lives were shortened by a revengeful act.

Revenge is the name of a TV show that aired from 2011 to 2015. The entire focus of the show was to see how much pain could be caused to the perpetrators of previously committed vile acts. While this may be a common modus operandi in virtually every culture of the world, indeed all of humanity—that does not make it a healthy response to our problems.

Forgiveness is a much more powerful response than revenge. It is harder to do initially but in the long run, the amount of energy spent, the time spent focusing on our previous pain, anger, and hate that eats at us, is far more consuming with revenge than it is with forgiveness.

True forgiveness stops the compulsive mentation that keeps the pain alive. It will not take away the memory, but it will allow the healing process to begin. Revenge keeps the wound open and seeping. Even in its completion, revenge does not heal. It only sets up another sorrowful mindset since a "good" person now feels "bad" for the action committed, even though the act was justified in that person's mind.

Forgiveness is freedom for the one who offers it. Forgiveness is not the same as absolution—if one commits an illegal act, they should be punished in a court of law. The "victim" of the act does not need to stay in bondage, by reliving the action through their hate, over, and over, and over. Forgiveness is not for the benefit of the perpetrator but for the benefit of the victim. In most cases, the perpetrators could care less if their victims forgive them or not. That is their problem to deal with in karmic payback.

The victims, however, can end their own pain by understanding that holding onto the thought is only prolonging their own suffering.

The actual words "I forgive you for ..." do not necessarily need to be spoken directly to the perpetrator. They can be expressed verbally just to oneself or to others, the forgiveness can be written down on paper (by hand) and then burned. It can also be a face-to-face conversation with the perpetrator. The point is to get it out of yourself and into the atmosphere where it can dissipate and no longer cause you suffering.

Exercise: Forgiveness—Part III

Exercise for allowing forgiveness to flow and eliminate the suffering.

Forgiving to Eliminate Suffering

1. Relax in a meditative posture, sitting upright.

2. Take three deep cleansing breaths.

3. Visualize the action that caused the pain.

4. Visualize and feel the heavy cloud of suffering and depression that hangs about you. Feel the weight of your anger. Feel the dampness of it in your lungs. Recognize how difficult it is to breathe because of the emotional shroud.

5. Be honest with yourself—what was your role? Unless it was a random act of violence or you were a young child at the time, visualize your role in the event. We always play a role in everything that happens to us.

6. Forgive yourself now. First, you have to forgive yourself for the part you played.

7. Forgive the other person for their actions. Make this sincere, from the heart forgiveness.

8. Visualize the shroud beginning to dissipate. Take some deep cleansing breaths—breathe in the universal life energy through the crown chakra (point at the crown of the head that connects us to the universal energy source) and convert it into love energy in the heart chakra. Use the converted heart energy to break up the shroud by visualizing releasing your breath through the heart chakra (point between the breasts through which our energetic body connects with the universal energy.) Once the shroud is gone, continue sending out heart energy to encase your entire being—all ethereal layers of your physical and spiritual bodies that extend out about 3-4 feet from your skin.

9. Keep filling the encasement with converted heart energy. Feel the healing properties of the heart energy. Allow it to fill in all of the holes in your being where the anger previously resided. Do you feel the difference? This is the energy you need for caring, not anger and hate.

10. Repeat the exercise whenever you feel yourself consumed by the anger to move the negativity out and allow the healing energy to soothe you.

Note: It may take several times repeating the exercise for the mentation to stop and for you to truly release the pain, but it will release. For your own health, do it.

How did you feel after completing the exercise the first time?

How did you feel after completing the exercise the second time?

How did you feel after completing the exercise the third time?

Continue tracking your progress. Repeat the process each time you get angry.

Painters' Pants

Most professions have their own standard code of dress. There is a range of acceptable dress depending on the occupation: casual street clothes, business casual, formal wear, or specific uniforms, like police or firefighters. The work clothes I find most interesting are worn by painters. Their white pants and shirts are covered with drops of various colors presenting a visual history of their work.

In a similar fashion, we all wear our own painters' clothes in life, some more visibly than others. Worry, stress, and happiness etch into our faces creating wrinkles and lines. If you study your face closely in a mirror, note the way your lines fall, you can read your own etchings.

Do the lines indicate frowning or smiling? Are they set in a grimace? Are your brows knitted together with a web of stress lines? Can you see lines of exhaustion? Hopefully, you see lines from smiling and laughing. Your face is a record of your past but also a canvas for the future.

Unless you have plastic surgery to tighten the sagging skin on your face, you cannot avoid facial wrinkles from developing as you age. Now is the time to determine if you want a permanent smile or frown to represent your life's experience.

When you change your frown to a smile, it is impossible not to change your accompanying attitude. At first, the smile may feel forced and disingenuous, but in a short period of time, the smile will trigger feelings of contentment and joy. It is hard to feel stressed out, angry, or fearful when you are smiling. So if you want a more joyful life that will reflect your historical record, start simple—smile. Smile at everyone you meet. Wear a smile always and you will find that the world will smile back at you.

Your "painter's" clothes will become richer, more pleasant and attain characteristics of trust, caring, and tenderness—and it all starts with a smile. One simple expression that costs you nothing can change your life for the better. ☺

Exercise: Mirror, Mirror on the Wall

Study your face closely in a mirror. Notice the way the lines travel across your face. Do the lines indicate frowning or smiling? Are they set in a grimace? Are your brows knitted together?

Change your expression into a smile. Are your lines changing direction?

Close your eyes and slow down your breathing, relaxing upon the exhale. Visualize all your stress and any negative tensions draining out of your body upon each exhale. After you feel your stress reduced, open your eyes and examine the lines in your face. Have they softened? The less stress you carry, the smoother your face will be.

Perform this exercise over a four-day period that covers at least two work days and two days you are off work. Pay attention to your stress level and facial expressions. Keep a log of when you catch yourself frowning; note your thoughts and feelings at the time of the event. Note when you are smiling, especially when you are not in conversation with another person. Record what you are thinking and feeling. Do you see repeating patterns that can be changed?

Part Two: Practices

Day 1. Expressions, Thoughts, and Feelings   Work _____   Off Work _____

Day 2. Expressions, Thoughts, and Feelings   Work _____   Off Work _____

Day 3. Expressions, Thoughts, and Feelings   Work _____   Off Work _____

Day 4. Expressions, Thoughts, and Feelings   Work _____   Off Work _____

Note the situations that routinely trigger frowns. Change your attitude about those situations. Welcome them into your life as learning experiences and smile in gratitude.

Continue to practice releasing your stress and relaxing your facial muscles. Practice your beautiful smile, lighting up the lives of others! Your smile may just eventually turn your frown lines upside down.

14 Release of Fear

Fear is the second ego trait and is the second layer in from the center. The location within the spiral provides a visual of how fear binds us. We cannot open inwardly or outwardly with fear; we are trapped. It has the ability to paralyze action, retard growth, deny happiness, and generally make our lives miserable. Fear is ego-based and rarely our friend in normal everyday existence.

Prevailing Winds

Life is most unpredictable. Yes, we may get out of bed the same time each day, go to the same workplace, and maybe even eat the same thing for lunch every day. However, what goes through our mind and how we interpret events changes—even if it is the same event from the day before.

How is it that we respond to stimuli diametrically opposite in manner and believe in the absolute fundamental correctness of both reactions or interpretations of the same event? EGO! The ego sees what it wants to see, hears what it wants to hear, and therefore believes that the two opposite conditions are both correct and subsequently believes they are both real. Well, they are very real in their personal reality.

Our ego has but one job, to protect the image of who we are. This protection extends to—protecting ourselves from ourselves. Oftentimes, it shields us longer—much longer, past the point when others know the truth about us before we know it ourselves.

At some point in our lives, we develop a mental image of who we are. We develop every detail, for example: we are a protector of our loved ones, we are forgiving, we are understanding, and we let others be who they want to be. We do not argue because we feel arguing is unhealthy, so we try to keep the relationship environment steady and peaceful. We love those in our lives unconditionally and take great pride in this fact because it shows our flexibility.

The character just described sounds like the perfect mate, perfect family person, and this is exactly right if the other mate has all the same (or most of the same) characteristics. However, if the other mate is controlling, a wounded ego that needs to lord over others to feel their own worth, then the first person described here becomes the victim of domestic abuse.

The abuse does not have to be physical to be damaging. In fact, the vast percentage of abuse in the United States is verbal, mental, or emotional in nature. Sometimes this can and does turn physical, but does not have to become physical to be effective. Because of the ego's inability to accurately read situations, it sees only what it needs to see to protect its image of itself. The ego willingly withstands great levels of pain rather than open its eyes to the truth.

So how do we break the cycle? How can we remove our veil of self-ignorance and pull back the shroud masking the mirror of our self?

The answer is mindfulness. When we live absolutely in the present moment, then we see each moment for exactly what it is without preconceived notions and judgments, only then we can see the truth. But we must set aside our emotions and preprogrammed thinking to do this.

In "active listening," we are taught to listen with an open mind to what another person is saying, and then take a moment to formulate a response after that person has finished speaking. This prevents us from making snap judgments before knowing all the details. Typically, we engage in non-active listening and while the other person is speaking, we stop listening and begin formulating our response.

Because of the magnificent complexity of the human mind, we are able to practice non-listening on ourselves. Our ego minds begin to interpret scenarios we find ourselves in as a way to protect us and not see what is really happening. Our "loved" ones standing before us yelling obscenities at us gets interpreted as "I must have done something to deserve this so I will have to try harder to get it right and please him or her."

This is classic abuser/victim mentality that keeps us rooted in behavior patterns that can (and often does) become deadly. By being mindful of each moment and not putting our protective ego overlay on the moment, we will be able to interpret events more accurately. But we must be willing to be completely honest with ourselves for the cycle to change. We have to drop our preconceived image we have of ourselves—it is usually wrong anyway, so why hang on to it?

Decide each moment on its own merit. When you do, you can better judge the prevailing winds and steer your actions to the proper course. Do not be afraid to steer in the opposite direction from past routes. If those routes brought you suffering in the past, don't go there, you will only get the same painful results.

Tell your ego to step aside and allow compassionate wisdom for yourself to shine through.

The flight attendant's instruction before takeoff is "Put on your own oxygen mask before helping others with theirs." This is applicable in all situations in life, not just when oxygen levels drop at 30,000 feet in the air. Inability to breathe at ground level has a debilitating effect too. So put on your mindful oxygen mask and leave it in place permanently. See what others see and put an end to your personal delusions. Abuse takes many forms, even the form of self-sabotage. No matter where it comes from, it is unhealthy, and must be eradicated with surgical precision.

Exercise: Assess your Relationships

Set aside a block of time when you are alone at home. Turn off your phone, radio, TV, any device that plays music, and computer games. Remove all distractions from the room in which you will work this exercise.

Assess the relationship with every person in your life that has significance. This includes those you live with, extended family if they are close, friends, and co-workers. Pretend that you are an outside observer making non-emotional, factual observations. When you write your notes on each person, write them from the point of view of this observer. Answer the following questions for each person. X refers to the other person; N refers to your name.

- Does X really listen to what N has to say and value N's opinions and thoughts? Does N really listen to what X has to say and value X's opinions and thoughts?

- Does X allow N to speak freely concerning issues that bother N about X without retribution? Does N reciprocate this freedom to X?

- Are X and N supportive of each other's creative endeavors, without mocking or destructive criticism?

- Is the relationship between X and N built and maintained on a foundation of healthy love and respect? Is the foundation instead maintained by fear used by either X or N?

- Does either X or N use money to control the other person?

- Does either X or N use guilt to control the other person?

- Does either X or N refuse to allow the other person to see friends or family members either with or without him/her? Is either one being cut off from outside support?

- Does either X or N tell lies about the other person to friends to gain sympathy for his or herself?

- Does either X or N ever raise his or her voice in anger to the other person? If so, how often? What are the typical reasons for the escalation?

- Has either X or N ever hit the other person or hit some other object or person (child) in a fit of rage?

- Does either X or N ever call the other person names like stupid, idiot, worthless, bitch, bastard, or other foul or derogatory insults? If so, how often?

- Does either X or N ever use children as a weapon against the other person? Has either told his/her child (ren) that the other parent does not love them, that only they love them?

Consider what advice you would give to a dear friend if any of your answers indicate a problem. Take that advice for yourself. If you cannot bear to act to protect yourself, get help from someone who can.

Setting Boundaries

As children, our parents are supposed to teach us how to make good decisions for ourselves. More often than not, they make the decision for the child and tell him or her "Do this because I said so." This of course, removes the opportunity to learn the decision-making process.

Many lower-level jobs are designed to remove the possibility of error by employees by having the administration make all the decisions and the worker bees carry them out. Unfortunately as we age, one's ability to make good decisions is assumed when this is not always the case.

When people have low self-esteem and self-love, their confidence in their own basic ability to make decisions can be shaken. They can be brilliant at what they do for a career choice, but in their personal lives, they are whipped around by more confident and manipulative people.

When they do seek out advice, which is typical since they don't trust their own ability, the advice should always be in the form of a learning opportunity. The Four Noble Truths (see Glossary) is the Buddhist decision-making tool that works wonderfully. By using this tool to walk them through the process and using the Eightfold Path and Six Perfections (see Glossary), you will not infringe on their free will to decide for themselves. Remember that just because they come to the "appropriate" decision, it does not mean they will act upon it at that moment.

When their own personal pain is unbearable, they will act. No one can move them until they are ready to move themselves. You can, however, be supportive during the process.

Is Competition Healthy?

As Americans, we are taught from a very young age to be competitive. Children as young as 4 and 5 years old are placed on T-ball and soccer ball teams. Competition in sports is a national pastime for every age group and oftentimes national sports teams provide regional identity and pride.

We are taught to be competitive in scholastics and on the job—to work harder and move ahead of our peers—to rise above them. At the same time, we are told we must work in teams cooperatively, but we are judged, evaluated, and rewarded as individuals. Being a "team player" is fine but not when it results in the promotion of another over you. It is not fair if another person gets credit for your effort.

On one level, competitiveness has served to help Americans to be highly motivated, innovative, and creative, but it has also fostered a dog-eat-dog culture. In many ways competition breeds fear—fear that we are not good enough, fear that others will pull ahead of us, fear that our weaknesses will be exposed. It also breeds discontent within us and fosters depression at the thought that we are less than, we are losers. We are not losers! We are not winners either. We are all just the same but playing roles that are not real. We see the roles as real but they are only masks that we wear. When we wear them long enough, they seem to become part of the psyche or essence of who we are. We begin to adopt the persona of a winner or a loser. This false view affects everything we do from that moment on.

If we see ourselves as losers, we stop trying to improve. Depression sets in. We may use drugs and alcohol to deaden our pain, but that behavior only increases it. We seek out others who feel the same way we do. If others are optimistic, we might try to bring them down to our level because "misery loves company." We are like the "Peanuts" comic strip character Pigpen, leaving soot on everything we touch.

If we believe ourselves to be winners, we may become overbearing, pretentious, and self-righteous. In time, we lose our friends and no one wants to be around us. This also can lead to depression. Again, we may use drugs and alcohol to deaden the pain, deaden the fear that maybe we are not truly "special." Maybe we are really just like everyone else. This concept in itself is painful for someone who was raised to believe that it is essential to rise above others.

How much simpler it would be for us to see the reality of things from birth—to never have the fallacy of rank imposed on us. What if we were taught that all people are equal in every way, shape, and form—not just giving the concept lip service because, as a democracy, we say everyone is equal? However, the actions of many do not support this theory. Can you imagine what a different society we could have if we all strived to act in support of equality?

I am not describing the failed Communist/Socialist ideal of the equality of the masses with the superior political power/dictator having supreme power. I am talking about real equality of everyone. If we believe that we are all equal and everyone goes through rough periods in their lives, then we are more willing to help each other. We become less likely to step on one another to move up higher. We are more likely to extend hands to each other, to support one another when we need it. Extending a hand is a sign of strength not weakness. By sharing that strength with another person, it only makes us stronger.

Consider whether you want to live in a society that is less fearful, less depressed, less addictive, less angry, and less directed. If you do, then it starts with you. You will need to reach out that hand of support to others. You will need to change your mindset and see yourself as equal to all others. You will need to treat others as you wish to be treated. You will need to let go of the fear of separation and ranking.

You also will need to see the reality that is before you—the reality of "Oneness." When you accept this as truth, your outlook and disposition will change. Your change will have a ripple effect on those around you and that ripple will then extend beyond those you touch.

Change begins with you. Releasing your fear to gain a more content existence and society, starts with you and me.

Exercise: Examine Your Fears

Consider your attitude towards mentoring others in your workplace. If your supervisor came to you and asked you to teach a new hire all you know about your job, what are the thoughts that immediately go through your head?

You are asked to work on a team by your employer. Everyone is asked to contribute new ideas for either problem solving or developing new products or services. You know that merit raises are awarded individually at the end of each year, and bonuses are given to the most productive employees each quarter. There is a finite amount of money for distribution so not everyone will receive a raise or bonus.

Does the reward system influence your willingness to bring new ideas to the communal table?

1) Always   2) Most of the time   3) Sometimes   4) Rarely   5) Never
6) Depends on who is on the team   7) Depends on whether the boss is in the room
Analyze your response.

Think about someone for whom you have great respect because of who they are, not how much money they have made. What are the characteristics you admire and aspire to emulate?

Do you exhibit those characteristics in your interactions with others?
1) Always   2) Most of the time   3) Sometimes   4) Rarely   5) Never

What personal behaviors can you change to emulate the person you admire?

Overcoming Fear

Winston Churchill famously said, "There is nothing to fear but fear itself." He was absolutely correct. Fear is an emotion that can retard your growth, stop you dead in your tracks, and prevent you from moving forward. Sometimes there may be a rational basis for the fear; for example, a friend has caught a contagious disease, so when you visit him at the hospital, you take precautions by wearing a mask and gloves for fear that you may catch the disease. This is fear, but it is also common sense.

Some of our fears are illogical, not based on common sense. Instead, they are based in our imagination, they are illusory. Our egos are afraid that they might not be successful at performing an act so they tell our brains that the act is harmful to us—they scream "Beware!" Other times, fear is a result of our not being able to stay in the present moment. We worry about what will happen in the future and the future, of course, is not yet written. We worry for the safety of our loved ones. We say we are concerned for them, but just maybe we are more concerned for ourselves. We may be concerned that our loved ones might be taken from us; if they die we will be alone.

Fear changes the chemistry of our brain. In the article, "Dealing with the Effect of Fear Anxieties," (The Appalachian) Nick Ianniello describes in detail the physiology of fear. The following is only a brief introduction:

> The physiological response to fear stimulus starts in the brain. The brain triggers the release of certain chemicals that cause the "flight or fight" response in human beings. This response is characterized by rapid heart rate, rapid breathing, flexed muscles, and an automatic focus on reacting physically. Once the chemicals released in the blood stream start to work, we are hardly aware of what is happening to us physically. We are simply in a reactive state controlled by the autonomic nervous system. All we want to do is run away from the fear agent or attack it directly. (Ianniello 2006)

Fear produces stress that also impairs our judgment. So how do we get our fear under control? We breathe. We stop, compose ourselves, close our eyes, and breathe mindfully. Mindful breathing is extremely relaxing.

Exercise: Mindful Breathing

There is no need to sit or be in any specific position for mindful breathing to be effective. You can do this driving or in a middle of an argument.

- Be silent and refocus your mind on your breath.

- Inhale from your diaphragm gently—you do not need to exaggerate the inhale.

- Visualize connecting with the calm energy of the universe through your crown chakra, at the top of your head.

- Visualize bringing in the white diamond light of the universe.

- Gently bring the light down your spine and let it flow to your feet.

- Exhale out of your mouth.

- Rest. Do not inhale again until your body compels you to do so. Do not force or exaggerate the exhale and pause, just rest.
- Repeat.

Continue to breathe mindfully until the thoughts or fears pass. Just relax.

15 Release of Prejudice

Prejudice is the third ego trait that causes us suffering. In many ways, prejudice is similar to fear. We pre-judge people and situations, make up stories about others, then convince ourselves that the story is true. Rarely is the story accurate and often the story portrays others in a less than favorable light. It is difficult to dispel our false beliefs once they have taken hold in our ego minds. Consequently, we may lose the opportunity to gain something valuable from the interaction.

Life is Easy

Some commonly used phrases about life, "Life is not supposed to be easy," "We're living on Easy Street," and "Living the life," can be misleading and contradictory. But one common phrase, "It is what it is," although it tends to be overused today by our youth, is absolutely accurate. "Life is what it is" and no more.

This phrase means that one should not be attached to the events in our lives because they are transitory. There should be no judgment as to the positive or negative aspect of events because everything is neutral. Once we label the events, we distort their very existence and worth as a learning tool on our path. If we call something "negative," then typically in our minds the event becomes of less value, something to shy away from, something to be ashamed of, or even something to hide or deny. If the event is "positive," we might not see it in its true form by giving it a more glowing aspect. It might play to our enlarged ego, our sense of whom we are, and distort that too. It may give us a sense of security, acceptance, or love that makes us feel better about ourselves or others. The interesting thing is that the exact same event can trigger all of these interpretations depending on how we color the event through our own biased eyes.

Another phrase, "I only believe what I can see," is really misleading because of the well-known phenomenon that a dozen witnesses seeing exactly the same event will each describe it differently. They also may interpret the meaning of the event a dozen different ways. So what is true and what is false? The short answer is that all of the various interpretations of the event are true and false. Each person's interpretation is true for him or herself but false for others. If this is the case, then clearly there are many "truths" resulting from one event; therefore, it would not be wise to become attached to any one of them.

When we accept an event as neutral, "it is what it is," and without judgment as to its positive or negative nature, we are better able to provide an authentic response. We are better able to learn what we are meant to learn from the incident and move on. It is the judgment that we place on something that keeps us attached to the events and to the results—results that change depending on our biased judgment.

Our subsequent actions can be very different depending on how we judge an event. Any action that we take based on that judgment will have a higher probability of being inappropriate when we are responding to our judgment rather than to the neutral event.

Instantly judging all that we see, do, and think is a very human response, however, it is what keeps us from living a stress-free life. It is impossible to shed stress if one minute we are being bullied one direction by feeling negative and the next minute being pushed another way feeling positive. Pretty soon, we have whiplash!

There is another common phrase, "Stay on the straight and narrow." The only way to do this is not to respond to our biased judgment of events. "It is what it is" and we should respond in an appropriate and authentic way.

One might criticize this suggestion with another common phrase, "You are taking the joy out of life" when the emotional roller coaster is berthed. This is a myth. You will find that your life will be much more joyful when you are on an even keel. You can better trust that the world you see around you is there for you to learn from, there for you to interact with, in stress-free intimacy.

Pavlov trained his dogs to respond in a certain way to repeated stimuli to obtain a reward of food or avoid a shock of electricity. When the rewards and punishments were removed, they still responded in the same way to the stimuli. Unfortunately, human behavior is entrenched in the same way. When we feel the rush of a high, or a strong emotional response due to positive or negative judgment of an event, we automatically know how to respond—because that is how we have trained ourselves to respond. To change our patterns in life, we have to change our response to events.

Life is not positive or negative, it is what it is, so we should deal with it and move on.

For example, Joe is sitting in a waiting area reading a magazine. Mike comes in and he is clearly agitated. Mike, who does not know Joe, growls something unintelligible to him. Joe could have several different responses.

1. Ignore it.

2. Interpret the remark as a personal affront, get upset, and challenge Mike with "What did you say to me!"

3. Become frightened and leave.

4. Feel sympathy for Mike because he is obviously distressed and say something to try to diffuse the situation.

All of these options, except the first, could provoke a dangerous response from Mike. No one knows why Mike is agitated so any judgment or interpretation on the part of Joe will most assuredly be wrong. Simply noting the events and staying alert for a possible potential second action that might put him in danger is the best course of action for Joe.

The agitation is not about anyone or anything in the waiting room. The event is related to Mike so why should Joe take it as his own stress? Merely noting it and letting it go is best. This is how to live a more stress-free life—note the events and let them go. Don't judge events; as soon as you do, you personalize them when 99.9 percent of the time the event has nothing to do with you. Don't you have enough stressors in your own life? Why take on the stressors of others?

"Life happens" and "it is what it is" and no more.

School Days Traumas

We all have a story about our elementary or high school experience. Maybe we have been bullied or were the perpetrators. Maybe we remember seeing the pain inflicted on some poor child who happened to be a bit different. The selected targets of bullies usually are a bit less than "perfect" in the eyes of the "in-crowd." They may be smaller or overweight, from a different ethnic background, or somewhat effeminate, have a speech impediment, or some mental or physical challenge. The experience felt by the targets can be devastating at the time and haunt them thereafter; but it doesn't have to scar the victim for life.

What is bullying? Psychologists will tell you that it is typically committed by children who themselves are victims of abuse in their homes but this does not account for the majority of the cases. Others are just plain acting out to get attention. Rene Veenstrain, et all in "Bullying and Victimization in Elementary Schools: A Comparison of Bullies, Victims, Bully/Victims, and Uninvolved Preadolescents" states:

> Bullies go for admiration, for status, for dominance unlike friendly teasing, bullying is long-term, unwanted and doesn't occur between social equals. Despite their

> aggressive behavior, bullies also want affection. Bullies care about the approval of their own in-group, so they strategically pick victims they know few other classmates will defend... Kids who are already socially awkward are more vulnerable to bullies. But there's no one thing that makes a child a target...For some kids, bullying behavior is just the tip of the iceberg. These children have other problems with aggression and control and may be abuse victims themselves. But there are also many otherwise well-adjusted children who just "think it's a cool thing to do." (679)

Is there something else going on here? The whole human experience seems to be based on the concept of ranking, knowing one's place in society. Class labeling starts at the moment of birth. We all fight those labels for the rest of our lives either to move up or maintain our status. Bullies are doing this. They are trying to determine or influence their place in the rank by inflicting pain on weaker members of the human tribe—survival of the fittest.

Parents of bullies almost always say, "I don't know why my child does that." Maybe they should look at the messages they are giving their children. Far too many of the religions preach that they are "the chosen ones"; that unless you follow their doctrine, you will be condemned for all eternity. Those who are the most fundamentally fervent are even more attached to this concept of superiority.

If you look at ethnic fighting and hatred around the world that has existed for centuries, it is striking that so much of the fighting was done, and continues to be done, in the name of God, Allah, or Yahweh. In every scenario, there is a battle of "chosen people" trying to impose their faith on others. Each side carries the wounds of centuries, of past transgressions, and they retaliate in a perpetual cycle. You hit me, so I hit you, back and forth, on and on.

What is interesting is that it is difficult to find examples where the Buddhists started a war. Certainly, Buddhists have been the targets of oppression but they are not the inflictors trying to force others to believe as they do.

Buddhists believe that ALL religions of the world are of value for those who get something spiritually uplifting from them. This concept of the "chosen one" does not come into play because everyone, without exception or exclusion, is "chosen." Everyone has Buddha-nature or life energy that comes from one and the same source.

If we teach our children from day one that we are all equal and that to hurt another would only cause pain to ourselves because we are connected, then children would be much less likely to strike out. Adults would be less likely to go to war.

Rank is an artificial construct developed by insecure minds that cannot accept or do not understand, the Buddhist teaching "Truth of Existence of All Things." This "Truth" states

Part Two: Practices

we are all interconnected and interdependent on all things and all things are equal. The word "things" here also includes all people.

Closely examine your own behavior, your words, the image you might project. Do you place yourself above or below others? When you encounter someone, do you mentally size them up and see where you think they are in comparison to yourself? This is wasted energy. The answer is always the same, we are equals.

Exercise: Self-Examination I

Day one: Pay close attention to your thoughts as you encounter people. Do you size them up? Do you rank yourself against your perception of them? Be honest with yourself; deluding yourself is of no use, it only delays your developmental process. This first day, merely observe your thoughts and record them here.

Day two: Observe your thoughts and subsequent behaviors based on those thoughts. Observe others reactions to your behaviors and record your observations here.

Day three: Actively work to control your thoughts and see everyone you encounter as equals. Pay attention to your behaviors and to the responses of others. Repeat this activity for several more days and record your progress.

Results: With earnest practice and attention, you will see your life change. You will see your relationships improve and you will feel better about yourself.

Keep practicing; see yourself and others without ranks, we are all equal. Your new attitude will change your life and the lives of those around you.

Prejudging Our Neighbors

Recently, I attended a meeting of a group of neighbors who wanted to form a neighborhood association. The goal is to be able to obtain funds from the city to improve the appearance of the neighborhood. The area was built in the 1940's and for most of that time, it has been a white middle-class neighborhood—a place for children to grow and the elderly to grow old. There are many apartment units in one end of the neighborhood. A few years after the owner of the apartments died, they became Section 8 housing; that is, subsidized by the government for low-income tenants. The residents now are primarily Hispanic, African American, and Middle Eastern Muslims.

The crime rate in the neighborhood has skyrocketed and the police are at the apartments daily. Drug deals are occurring on the street corners. Fear has replaced friendliness.

At the meeting, the newly formed association was approving the by-laws written by a committee. Many people wanted only homeowners to be eligible for membership. One person wanted "homeowners" to be in the name of the organization. The group wanted to exclude all apartment dwellers. One person spoke up and challenged the group. She said, "Maybe if we invite the apartment residents to join us, they will feel more like part of the neighborhood and feel more welcome. There are poor families living among us that are trying to get ahead. Why not extend a friendly hand to include them. It is wrong to write a charter based on exclusivity instead of inclusivity."

After a lot of emotionally charged discussion it was agreed that anyone could join but to sit on the executive committee you had to be a "resident" (not necessarily a homeowner) for one year.

This meeting was a perfect example of how people presume to know what is in the minds and hearts of others. They assumed all of the apartment dwellers were troublemakers by associating them with a single factor—living in troubled low-income housing.

This may be a Pollyannaish view of the situation, but maybe if people feel included, if they feel welcomed, if they feel valued as neighbors and humans, then the neighborhood would change. Of course, there are some people who will continue to break the law, but the vast majority of them just want to live in peace and provide a better life for their families. Prejudging people only serves to keep us in our own cell made of fear. We construct the bars ourselves with our fears, hatred, and ideas of self-superiority.

We do not live on independent islands. We live together. We provide each other opportunities to learn lessons and grow. Without our interaction with those who are different, we would become stagnant. Including all residents in our association will stabilize the neighborhood. Including people who do not look like us in our group of friends and colleagues will stabilize our work places. Including others who are different into our lives will stabilize our country. Including others of different cultures as valued people will stabilize the planet. It all begins with making NO assumptions about others. It begins with inclusionary not exclusionary attitudes and behaviors. It begins with recognizing that we are all one. Each of us has our own script to follow in this play of life. Our characters do and must interact. There is only one play. See all others as important characters in this play, the climax of which is peace, understanding, and personal growth for us all, individually and together.

Exercise: Reach Out

Activities to Expand Your Circle

Focus on finding common ground and learning about different ideas and habits.

- Take a walk around the neighborhood and make a point of talking to several people who don't look like you or sound like you. Strike up a real conversation, not just say "hi" in passing.
- Invite someone from work or the neighborhood to a cookout. Get to know them on a personal level.

- Join a book club at your central library in a downtown area.
- Volunteer for a community clean up activity.
- Volunteer at Habitat for Humanity.
- Join a neighborhood garden or start one yourself.
- Get involved with your neighborhood association or start one yourself.
- Volunteer at an agency for the mentally or physically disabled.
- Volunteer at an elementary school reading program or a literacy program for adults.
- Join a Silver Sneakers group at your local YMCA and participate in their group activities.
- Get involved with an activist group championing a cause promoting equality for minorities, clean environment, elimination of corruption in government, or any other group that attracts you.
- Join a church group, drum circle, meditation group, or any other group of interest that moves you into contact with a diverse group of people and make new friends.
- Join an interfaith group.

Journal your progress:

- What went through your mind at your first outing?
- What conversation starters did you use? Were they effective? If not, what can you say differently the next time?
- How long did it take you to feel at ease? (Track this over time.)
- How many different people did you engage in conversation?
- How comfortable were you in speaking with new people?
- What commonalities did you discover?
- What new ideas did you discover?
- What will you try next time?

16 Release of Separation

Separation is the fourth layer of the spiral and last of the ego traits that cause us suffering. This trait, more than the other three, is more likely to lead to depression and suicide.

There are over seven billion people living on the planet. There are not seven billion plus separate and distinct individuals; at our core, we are all one. We are all part of the same whole, which also includes animal, plant, and earth energies. Cultures that are highly individualistic and promote a strong sense of personal individualism, competition, societal ranking, and that are based on material acquisition have more problems accepting this truth than collective cultures. Collective cultures that promote living in harmony with nature, group cohesion, dependency, and cooperation over competition, individual rights, and class superiority are better able to understand the interconnectedness of all beings.

Which Religion Gets it Right?

Religion has existed ever since man began to walk upright and have a language that could be used to form independent thoughts. The belief systems were as varied as the number of cultural groups. Around the globe today, there are hundreds of religions that believe they have the true understanding of faith.

Which one is correct? The truth is that all are correct—in their own way for their own people. Does it matter that we all do not believe the same thing? No, it does not matter at all.

It is the core of our beliefs that is critical for humanity to survive together. That central core IS the same: recognition of a higher power or universal energy and respect your fellow man. The rest of the rules are just trappings to control the behaviors and thoughts of the followers.

Do not fear to be free. Free to believe only that which makes sense to you in your heart. Beware of greed, ego, and fear that blind us to the truth and color our interpretation of truth, which affects our decisions

The ego-made belief that one religion is more perfect than another, or that specific adherents are the "chosen ones," is dangerous. The belief that people must follow a prescribed activity to be happy for eternity after the physical body has died is dangerous. One needs only to turn on the radio and listen to the news about suicide bombings and religious martyrdom to know this is true. This erroneous belief in exclusivity has caused more suffering and death since the dawn of man than any other belief.

It is time to stop the lies and change the dialogue. Remove the obstacle of prejudice from your eyes and see the truth. Every human is formed exactly the same. We are all born with the same number of organs. We walk upright, not slithering on our bellies. We all have brains to think and hearts to modify the thoughts of the brain. Outward appearances are just ways of distinguishing family groupings, no different than the unique stripe patterns of zebras so that the young can find their mothers in the herd.

The "enemy" is not one who looks or believes differently. The enemy is the lie that tells us we are different. Remove the lie and the world lives in peace and harmony. It is that simple.

- We are one, not many.
- We are the same, not distinct.
- We are forever joined as one—in the past, in the present and in the future.
- Killing another human being is the same as cutting off a part of yourself. The repercussions ripple throughout the human herd.

So what can one individual person do? Change your view of separateness into one of commonality. Your behavior and thought patterns will naturally change too. If you change your view, you will influence others around you to change their views. Eventually, like dominos, we will all lie touching one other in the connected chain that we are.

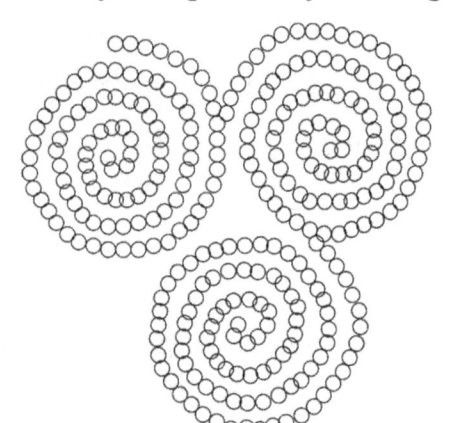

Be brave. Change your view. Start the dominos falling within your circle of influence. Your circle will affect other circles, which will affect even more. Peace is possible if we change our view. We are one, not many.

Exercise: All the Same

Activities to try:

- Take a class at your community college on world religions.
- Check out a library book on world religions and read it with an open mind.
- Visit churches of various faiths and talk to the ministers.
- Join an interfaith group.
- Celebrate high holidays with your coworkers of different faiths.

Journal your findings:

- What are commonalities with your own religious tradition?
- What are customs that you find interesting?

- Do you accept that their beliefs are right and valid for them just as your beliefs are right and valid for you?

Dance for Your Life

Today I witnessed an amazing contemporary dance production. The dancers exhibited extremely high energy. They gave 100 percent of themselves. They did not just show up for the performance, they lived it, they became it, it popped with excitement and drew the audience into their story.

This is how we should live our lives; not as mere observers, never being brave enough to jump whole-heartedly into the role. We all know people that seem just to sit on the sidelines and watch. They are fearful of taking risks. They need to know the outcome of things—or at least have a pretty good idea of how things will unfold before they move into action. Surprises are unwelcome, even good surprises, because they feel a loss of control.

The beauty of the performance lies in not knowing what the dancers were going to do next. Would the tempo pick up or slow down? Maybe they would slide on the floor or maybe they would do my favorite move and fly though the air, leaping like a gazelle. Regardless of the moves, they were all beautiful.

What made it really spectacular was the interaction of the performers. The solo routines were delightful, but certainly not as captivating as watching the whole troupe depend on each other, to be there to swing together, or catch one another in the air, or set in motion a wave action—the interplay was spellbinding.

Thus, it is in life, too. We can be, and are at times, individual performers in our lives. We have to take school exams by ourselves; however, for the most part, everything else in life is enhanced when we involve others. Collaboration, sharing, supporting, playing off other's performances—this is what makes life more interesting but less controlled.

If I do something completely by myself, I perceive that I will control the outcome, and therefore it will be an outcome with which I will be comfortable. My problem-solving skills are restrained by my own field of experience and will therefore be less creative. I may never be able to come up with a workable solution.

Instead, when we involve others, when we ask for help, we are able to draw on their experiences, and combined with ours, we can create something completely different. To be able to do this, we have to squelch our egos. We have to admit that we do not know how to do something. This is an unconscionable thing to do for those who must have total control in their lives at all times.

Fear of the unknown and our own perceptions of whom we are (ego-based), keeps us on the sidelines of life. A perfect solution is like a seed that is planted in fertile soil (material world). It is watered with opportunities to grow. The seed sprouts and blossoms, but without pollination of the blossom from a bee, it cannot reproduce. We need pollination from others in our own lives. Even the hermit in a dense forest needs interaction with birds and animals upon which to draw inspiration for solving problems.

We are social beings by our very nature, designed to work together. We need to trust that others will "have our backs." We need to trust that the best solution will only come from giving up control of the minuscule. Once we accept the support and guidance of others, the path becomes easier for us. We do not have to reinvent the wheel; we can build upon the experiences of others.

Your ability to control the outcomes of all events in your life is a myth anyway; it is only an illusion. So if it is not real, then why put all of your energy into trying to control things you cannot? It is like being on a raft in the middle of a fast moving river. You can paddle with all your strength to try to remain in the exact same place but you cannot maintain it for long, so why try? Instead, go with the flow. Allow yourself to be transported and supported by others. You can ride their waves and still make it your own experience.

Exercise: Ask or Tell

Day one: Rarely do we realize that we tell people to do things instead of asking them. For one day, pay close attention to how you talk to others. Do you preface your statements with "Will you please…" or just state a command? Even if you give the command in a normal speaking tone, a command is still interpreted as a command. Document and classify the types of statements you make. Notice and document the response from others to the different types of statements. Pay close attention to how you speak to family members. We are more likely to command family than others.

Part Two: Practices

Day two: Make a conscious effort to convert all commands into requests. Document your efforts and the responses you receive.

Day three: Continue your efforts to make only requests instead of demands. Is there someone with whom this exercise is more difficult than others? Analyze the underlying reason for this difference.

Beyond: Remove all commands from your way of speaking. Commands are only appropriate in emergency situations to protect others from harm.

The Value of One Life

In today's entertainment world, the cost of one life isn't worth much. Every second of every day, you can turn on the TV or scan movies and see someone blown away. The higher the level of violence, the bigger the attraction. Why is this?

We humans are the only species that kill one another for sport, for pleasure, or for no reason at all, just because we can. What then is the value of life? Non-human life is worth even less than human. Cruelty to animals is against the law, but killing them is not. Why not?

If we are going to advance in our level of "civilization," we need to take many steps backward to a time when animals and man were of equal value. Animals have always been part of the food chain, but they were blessed and thanked for their ultimate contribution. The one killed and the consumer both realized the ultimate sacrifices made for humans.

So again, I ask, what is the value of one life?

Consider the honeybees; they are becoming extinct through interbreeding with the aggressive African bee. In many regions, bees no longer pollinate our crops to the degree they once did. The world's food supply has dwindled as a direct result of this loss. Humanity is dependent on a "lowly" honey bee.

Every time a human is killed, his or her death provides opportunity for growth; teaching others what not to do if they want to stay alive. However, in our eye-for-an-eye, or more realistically, eye-for-a-hundred-eyes world, the only lesson is revenge. Revenge are acts of manipulative payback; the more painful the retribution, the better. If anyone is caught in the way as collateral damage, well it so be it.

Why? What is the point? We have heaped so much pain upon each other over the period of the existence of man that it no longer has shock value; except that more is better. Our spiral into self-destruction and taking the rest of the animal and plant kingdoms with us has to stop, or at least slow down.

How can we do this? We change by recognizing the undeniable interconnection, direct linkage, of all sentient beings. All religions of the world pay lip service to this reality. They all have rules that command against killing but why do so many of the faithful enjoy films, books, and video games depicting incredible brutality against men, women, and children?

The change can start—needs to start—with you. Turn off the violence by refusing to be entertained by it. Refuse to financially support the continued chaos that encompasses our every sensation. Turn off the news on the radio, TV, Internet, and in print. Turn it all off.

Celebrate positive connections, helping one another, nurturing each other, and supporting all sentient beings.

So I ask one last time—what is the cost of one life? Answer—there is no quantifiable value; it is invaluable. Without the linkage of lives, we all perish. We need to be the role models for others, modeling compassion, love, and support. Stop the craziness! How?

Exercise: The Value of Life

1. Be shocked again by violence. Be repulsed, not entertained by it.

2. If you do not pay money to view films, watch TV shows, pay/play video games, or purchase/read books that depict and glorify violence, then the genre will cease to dominate our entertainment culture.

3. You can write letters to newspapers, directors, producers, magazines, and bloggers demanding more wholesome entertainment. Demand the return of real comedy, not just sex farces.

4. In your sphere of influence, you can convince others that revenge is unacceptable.

5. Devalue the "strong" over the "weak." We all have both characteristics in us.

6. You can speak out against violence, both real and for "entertainment." Passive acceptance can be considered the same as doing it yourself.

7. Truly believe and realize the interconnection of all, in the intricate self-supporting chain of life. When one link is removed prematurely by force, all are affected.

8. Generate positive and loving thoughts; send them to yourself, your family, friends, and most importantly to your enemies.

9. Turn your enemies into your friends by accepting their different ideology as okay for them. Focus on those areas where you can find common ground and agreement. It is possible to get along with someone who thinks differently than you.

We arc all bees.

Abandonment

Why do so many of us have fears of abandonment? We fear that others will leave us. The psychologists tell us that this fear typically stems from an incident in childhood in which we perceived that a loved one left us. Maybe a parent died or, as a result of a divorce, a parent became unavailable. Sometimes it occurs early in our young courtship experience, when a budding love fails to produce the desired blossoms, and we feel let down and rejected. Regardless of when the seed was planted, typically it is watered with fear over the years until the potential threat of someone leaving us becomes stronger than the potential bond of love for and by another.

This fear of being abandoned becomes a self-fulfilling prophecy. Once we believe that all loving relationships will end with the other person leaving, it is the job of our egos to make us right.

A couple of different behavioral patterns may develop. First, we tend to put one foot into a new relationship and keep one out, just in case we need to pull back in a hurry to protect our hearts. This means we are never fully present and available to grow a new relationship. It is like watering a newly planted seed, and once it begins to sprout we stop watering it and expect the plant to survive in dry soil. Of course, we also tell the plant "If you really love me you will grow without water." Clearly, this is a self-defeating strategy.

Another typical behavioral pattern is to be the first to pull back from the relationship, thereby sparing oneself the pain of being left behind. Often, the other person incorrectly identifies this behavior as a difficulty in making commitments, when in fact it is just the opposite. We want very much to make that commitment but fear that we are the only ones really invested in it, so we "protect" our hearts and pull back first. Later in life, this influence can even cause us to punish our grown children when they leave the nest. When they return for special occasions, we make subtle (or not so subtle) mean comments to them; this serves to ensure a reduction of visits in the future. It also causes the adult child to feel as if they have to be very careful about what they say and do, lest they are showered with fear disguised as anger.

Obviously, according to the law of cause and effect, we are setting ourselves up to validate our fears. We need to be right, even at the cost of our own happiness.

So how can we stop the self-sabotage? The first step is to realize that we are never alone. It may seem as though we are alone, but in fact this in not the case. When the "Go Away" signs are removed from our hearts, and replaced with "Welcome, happy you are here!" things will change. When fear is replaced by gratitude, when anger is replaced by generosity, when withdrawal is replaced by commitment to serve, a new person emerges. The new person becomes a beacon of light that naturally draws others in.

It is impossible to be absolutely alone. Even if you go off into a jungle and live by foraging in the forest, there are still other life forms with which you will interact. It is also impossible to cut the energetic ties of the universe that binds us to every other person. Once we change our attitudes about who we are from "I'm not worthy so everyone will leave me "to "I want to support others and I am grateful for everyone and everything in my life"—our lives change.

We are fully in control of how our own seeds will grow and blossom. If we water them with fear of rejection, they will be stunted. If we water them with gratitude, they will grow into something quite extraordinary. The scent and beauty of mature plants or relationships will strengthen the mutual support that is necessary for them to endure.

Gratitude is a behavioral pattern that, when developed and entrained, will directly change the course of cause and effect sequences, from self-defeating to all-embracing. Gratitude is the water that, when applied liberally, allows all life to flourish.

War Mindset

Every country has its national holidays. Some are tied to celebrations of the outcome of a war with another nation to establish its independence. There is also typically a day of mourning for those who died defending their country.

War spawns much hatred and disease of the mind, body, and spirit. In some political parties, war is glorified, a rallying point for nationalistic fervor. It is seen as positive precisely because it pushes people into supporting one specific agenda or party. It fires up people to hate everyone that is not just like them.

On a spiritual growth scale, this behavior ranks pretty low. All war is bad; it is nothing other than the clash of egos. One person or group believes they are superior to another. War also is typically about greed and domination.

What if we had a global society that did not glorify war but instead glorified peace; what would the world look like? If video games of war were replaced with games of helping others instead of killing them, the mindset of the players would be molded differently. If young children were taught to play with construction blocks instead of toy weapons and soldiers, the world could have more projects where people worked together to solve problems instead of killing.

If you think about it, the common early developmental activities in the United States is to train young boys to be soldiers, to fight, to dominate. Why are we surprised, when as adults, that is what many males want to do—fight and dominate?

Now you will say, "If we didn't train them early, then we would have no one willing to go to war, to give their lives to defend our nation and our people against aggressors." This is true, but if in every nation of the world, the children were taught to play at peaceful coexistence instead of war then we would not need to fear attacks on our borders.

So where am I going with this very old argument that has been preached by pacifists for centuries without making an impact? The principle of "no self" is the key. We are all one. We are connected. We are all part of the same whole. If you kill another, you damage yourself—a part of you dies too.

Recently, I was speaking with a veteran and he told me his first "kill" was a young boy. The child had explosives attached to him and he was sent in to be a human bomb. The vet talked of his struggle to pull the trigger, he eventually did, but the horror of the event still haunts him more than 20 years later. Part of him died that day with the child.

We do have a choice in how we see the world, and how we see the world affects how we behave. If every human on the planet realized and accepted the fact that we are all equal, that we are all one, that peaceful coexistence is better than domination, everyone would be happier and healthier.

For this to happen, the mindset change has to start with you and me. We have to exemplify the behavior of acceptance. We have to model the truth of unity and sameness. We have to train our children very early on and consistently throughout their lives to recognize the oneness of all.

One stone dropped into a lake has a ripple effect in the entire body of water. One change in your attitude and in mine, will change our behaviors, which in turn will cause a ripple effect in the sea of humanity.

Now is the time to change, before another life is ended needlessly. You, me, him, her, they—we are all one.

Garage Sales

Most people have been to at least one garage sale at some time in their lives. Perhaps you have even held one yourself to clear out unwanted items and clutter from your home. Such sales are interesting analogies for life in general. You go through your home collecting odds and ends that have lost their utility and meaning for you. Then you try to sell them to someone else to squeeze the last bit of value out of each one.

The potential buyers are interesting as well. There are those that show up before the appointed start time to catch you off guard and try to obtain the highest quality items for less than the posted price. Often these people will then turn around and immediately sell the same items for several times more what they paid.

Don't we sometimes do this ourselves in other situations? We might try to skirt the rules and get something for less. This is a "seller beware" mentality. Of course the opposite "buyer beware" mentality exists, too. Either way, the behavior, although it might not be illegal, is also not spiritually pure.

What is the difference between ethical behavior and spiritually pure behavior? Every business course or book has an ethics chapter dealing with how one should behave in that specific discipline. The problem is that the recommended course of action is designed to keep the practitioner and company out of jail, not to do what is in the highest good.

"Do no harm" is a common stance. While this is commendable, it does not go far enough. "Do the highest good" is much better for the life and cohesion of the planet. This reflects spiritually pure action.

Individual and institutional egos encourage employees to get the most they can out of a potential sale—again "buyer beware." Many will justify these actions as "It is just business, what you have to do to be successful." Is this really true?

Win-lose transactions are just that; one side rises at the expense of the other. This is NEVER healthy for either side. This is true for business and it is true for relationships in our private lives.

When we extend our hand to help rather than trick, pull people up with us, instead of stepping on them to get to the top, then we all win. Ultimately, this is the best scenario.

Unfortunately, you often hear the arguments "It is not my responsibility to care for others." "The only responsibility a company has is to make money for its investors." These views are more than just shallow, they are dangerous.

They are dangerous to the ones who hold the view because it hardens their hearts to the plight of others. The "others" are actually extensions of themselves, ourselves, since we are all part of the same whole. So in reality, when we take advantage of someone else, we are only harming ourselves.

I realize that those who practice win-lose behaviors do not buy this argument. It is hard to understand it when they are living in their mansions, driving fine cars and consuming the highest quality of everything, while the "others" are out of sight and out of mind.

I encourage everyone to spend time helping out in a soup kitchen or visiting poor neighborhoods to see the direct impact of greed and disadvantage. Hopefully, the experience will trigger an awakening of consciousness in many individuals that will move a small step forward toward healing the planet.

Part Two: Practices

Exercise: Ethical Guidelines

Below is a chart of various types of ethical philosophies that are typically taught in a college course on ethics. The definitions are modified to make sense on a personal level. Read through them and in the third column, rate on a scale of 1-5, each philosophy as to whether you believe that style is in the greatest good for all humanity. Number 1 is the highest good, and 5 is the most selfish. Then, in the fourth column, rate each based on how you live your life. Number 1 is most like you, and 5 is least like you. Do not rate them based on what you believe about yourself, but instead on what you do. No one else is going to see your answers so be completely honest with yourself. All views are legal. You may rate multiple views as a one; often we hold more than one ethical philosophy.

Theory	Definition	Rate 1-5 (1 is in the highest good)	Rate 1-5 (1 is most like you)
Egoism	An ethical system defining acceptable behavior as that which maximizes consequences for the individual – what is best for you is what is right.		
Utilitarian	The moral worth of actions or practices is determined by their consequences. Actions are desirable if they lead to the best possible balance of good consequences over bad consequences. The greatest good for the greatest number of people should be the overriding concern of decision makers.		
Friedman Doctrine	The only social responsibility of business (and our own earning potential) is to increase profits, so long as we stay within the rules of law.		
Cultural Relativism	Ethics are culturally determined and we should adopt the ethics of the cultures in which we operate; "when in Rome, do as the Romans do."		
Righteous Moralist	If my personal ethics are appropriate for me at home then they are appropriate everywhere even if they violate the spirit of the law elsewhere.		
Naïve Immoralist	Actions are ethically justified if everyone else is doing the same thing. If everyone else is behaving questionably then it is OK for me to do the same.		

Part Two: Practices

Theory	Definition	Rate 1-5 (1 is in the highest good)	Rate 1-5 (1 is most like you)
Kantian	People should be treated as ends and never purely as means to the ends of others. People have dignity and need to be respected, they are not machines.		
Rights Theories	Fundamental human rights form the basis for the moral compass by which one should navigate. There are basic principles that should always be adhered to irrespective of culture.		
Justice Theories	Focus on the attainment of a just distribution (one that is considered fair and equitable) of economic goods and services. All economic goods and services should be distributed equally except when an unequal distribution would work to everyone's advantage.		

(Chart is an adaptation of material from Hill 143-150)

If there is a disconnect between what you believe to be in the highest good and how you behave, analyze your behavior and see what you can improve.

17 Acknowledging Acceptance

Acceptance is the first of the spiritual traits and is the fifth layer of the spiral. What you are encouraged to "accept" is that everything happens for a reason. If you accept this premise, then everything in life is no more than a learning opportunity, an opportunity to improve yourself and reduce your suffering. Once you learn the intended lesson, then you will be able to take judicious steps to change and improve your condition.

Bone Spurs

(This story is not intended to give medical advice; it is an analogy for troubles in life. If you have a medical condition, please see a medical professional.)

Pain is interesting. It can come and go for no apparent reason. Take the pain of a bone spur on your heel. You can wake up one morning and not be able to put weight on your heel without feeling like a dagger is trying to come through your skin. So what do you do? You walk on the ball of your foot to avoid putting pressure on your heel. After a couple of hours or a day, the pain will subside by itself—maybe.

If not, there are three solutions to the problem of the bone spur:

1. Surgery to eliminate the bone spur.
2. Bed rest, or at least staying off your foot, and elevating the heel for a period of time.
3. Do nothing and ignore it. Put on a cushioned shoe and get on with life. Just work through the pain.

Which solution would you select? The first option—surgery to cut out the offending bone spur? In life, you always have the choice of responding to painful events in this way. You can take some anesthesia, alcohol, or drugs, and hope someone will remove the source of the pain. Rarely does this result in a real solution to the problem and the use of the anesthesia may complicate the issue.

The second option is to do nothing and elevate the foot, relax on bed rest. This one is often coupled with the use of anesthesia to stop the throbbing pain. While in bed, you read, watch TV, play computer games, and such to divert your attention from what is really going on. Yes, eventually this solution will work, but it is only a temporary fix and will come back to haunt you over and over until you address the problem in earnest.

The third option is to continue walking on the foot and work through the pain. This solution is the most difficult but the results are better. You don't rely on someone else to fix it for you and you don't avoid it. You deal with the issue head on and work through it. The solution typically takes longer to obtain results. When you select it and actively work it, other issues may also crop up along the way. Once you understand the problem and release it, the pain is either completely eliminated or dramatically reduced. The next time it occurs, it is easier to deal with.

Virtually, all of the pain we face in life comes with these three potential solutions. The one we select is often based on the amount of strength and courage we have at that particular moment in time. We will only select the third option after repeatedly being presented with the problem and it appears that if we don't, it will just keep coming back.

So why do we subject ourselves to the endless cycle of pain? Clearly, it is much better in the long run to just deal with problems as they arise the first time. Work it out and move on. Draw on your inner strength. Stand before a mirror so that you can get the full image of the problem. If you need some help, instead of a surgeon, see a counselor or spiritual guide to help you to understand the root of the problem. Don't waste time, money, and false hope that someone else can fix you. Only you can fix yourself but a shoulder to support you along the way can help you to make better choices in your own care.

You may also need a period of bed rest but do not use it as a diversionary tactic. Instead, use the time to regroup and to reflect, to gain personal strength, then attack the problem with a renewed sense of purpose, and then all will be revealed.

Exercise: Self-Examination II

We all have reoccurring problems that we face time and time again. Think back over your life as far as you can remember. What issue (or two) keeps coming up for you? The issue does not have to be something major like 10 divorces; it can be seemingly small like an inability to get to appointments on time, not picking up after yourself, starting projects but not finishing them, etc. What do others nag you about?

List all of your behaviors and mindsets that could use improvement.

Analyze each of the items you listed without beating yourself up. Look at them objectively. Then write a couple of suggestions as to how you can change each pattern. Really try to get to the root of each behavior. Examples: Maybe the behavior is a defense tactic; if so, what are you afraid of? Maybe it's just laziness; if so, how can you generate enough energy to fix it? Maybe it is a learned pattern from your parents; how can you break that pattern? Maybe the behavior is not important to you, but it's irritating or inconvenient to others; how can you convince yourself to put the needs of others first?

Happy Birthday

Birthdays are wonderful times in our lives and they are gifts that occur each year. These are opportunities that are given to us to renew our connection and recognition of who we are—at our core. Birthdays are opportunities to express gratitude to our ancestors and those in our lives that provide us with opportunities for growth on a daily basis.

Oftentimes, they are periods of reflection. "I am one year older and one year closer to dying. What have I done with my life thus far? What should I do with my life in the future?" This reflection can be a celebration if you are satisfied or a lamentation if you feel there is much room for improvement.

The good news is that in respect to your past, there should be no regrets whatsoever. You did what you did; you thought what you thought because of where you were in your growth cycle—PERIOD. You needed those past events to occur to learn what you needed to learn—as painful as it might have been. Your future has yet to be written. It can be whatever you choose to make it. I'm not referring to material gain, which has nothing to do with happiness and growth on your path. In fact, it can be an impediment if you get caught up in the myth that the material world can satisfy your needs—it cannot.

You need ONLY yourself to be happy. If you cannot find a way to be happy with yourself alone, then no number of other people can help. Your loving children and spouse certainly are wonderful fringe benefits, but if you don't love yourself, if you are not comfortable in your own skin, then it doesn't matter that they are in your life.

So take this day of rebirth and renewal to heart. Don't use it merely as an opportunity to imbibe in spirits of the liquid kind but instead drink in the spiritual energy and wisdom of the universe, earth, and sages. Spend some time in quiet reflection. Truly be grateful for your life as it has been up until now. Rejoice in the continued opportunity to grow and develop your spiritual self on your pathway to enlightenment. Today is truly a gift. Thank your parents who enabled you to be in your physical form. Thank them for providing direction and protection as needed.

Life is wondrous. Live it to the fullest spiritually. Love yourself and others will love you too. Turn everyday into a birthday. For every day, every moment is an opportunity for renewal and reflection. Rejoice! Happy birthday, today and everyday!

Exercise: Self-Examination Meditation

After completing the previous exercise, Self-Examination II, take a few moments to visualize a new you:

1. Find a comfortable place to relax in an upright position. If it has been awhile since you completed Self-Examination II (page 71), reread what you wrote.

2. Begin Mindful Breathing (go back to the exercise on Mindful Breathing and review page 48). Normal inhale, normal exhale, then relax and pause, breathe in this pattern throughout the exercise.

3. Visualize before you two versions of yourself—side A and side B. Side A is your old self with all of the flaws of the past. Side A has a gray shroud covering it. Side B is your new self, the one you would like to become. Side B is radiant with light beaming from it on all sides.

4. On the inhale, visualize B breathing in light and energy through the crown chakra, bringing it down to the heart chakra. On the exhale, send the light out of the heart of B into the heart of A.

5. Keep repeating step 4 until A is as bright as B, washing away the shroud.

6. Then visualize B encouraging A to be the best he/she can be. Tell A that there is no reason to feel guilty, that together you will move into the future as a renewed and empowered being.

7. Visualize B hugging A, the light becoming brighter as the two sides become one.

8. Relax and feel complete.

18 Acknowledging Compassion

Compassion is the second spiritual trait and the sixth layer of the spiral. Simply stated, compassion is the personal desire for all beings to be free of suffering and live a life of joy, not just oneself. It then follows that one's actions and behaviors reflect this desire. Those actions purposefully help to improve the lives of others.

Ego Control and Finding Your Way

Sometimes even accomplished people need direction. The problem is, those are the people that are least likely to realize they need guidance and are the ones less likely to accept it. Guidance comes in many forms. When it comes as a thought that just "appears" in our own heads, it is easy to accept because we believe it comes from us. Rarely is that the case. Guides/buddha's/angels are at work. This type of guidance is very common but rarely do we recognize it as guidance.

Another type of guidance comes from our friends/families/peers. If the guidance is presented in the form of a story, "That happened to me and this is how I responded, and this was the favorable outcome," then we might listen. If the guidance is presented as "Do this. This is what I did and it worked." If the other person is acting in a loving and caring way, then we might listen if we believed the other person really has our best interest at heart.

The third kind of guidance comes from an authority figure—there are many sorts of these. If the guidance comes across as compassionate, we may listen. If it comes as a command—forget it. The guidance will instead be seen as intrusive, unwarranted, and unwanted. The human ego reacts by pushing back: "Who are you to know what is best for me?" Unfortunately, it is often this very advice that is most helpful for us. The big question is how do you silence the ego long enough to hear and learn?

Another question that often comes up is "Is this person just trying to take over and dominate the situation? How do I know that his or her intentions are positive for me? Am I being manipulated?" These are normal reactions but not helpful ones.

Before deciding on issues of importance, meditate on these questions:

1. What action or decision is in my highest good?
2. What decision or action is in the highest good of others?

Be open to receiving messages, you do not have to answer these questions alone.

So what do you do if the responses for these questions are opposites? Is there a middle ground? More often than not, the answer to the second question will be the correct answer. Dealing with your own egos and putting the good of others first is very difficult.

Consider this story:

There are some birds of different species hanging around. They are soaring on the wind, playing in the thermals, and just enjoying being birds. Below them, they see a younger bird that is in the thermal for the first time, trying to get the hang of how to glide with the energy of the wind. The younger bird flies too close to the ground and a coyote appears from nowhere and snaps at it.

The young bird freaks out and the rest of the birds scatter out of harm's way—all but one. This one brave bird swoops down and heads directly for the coyote, scaring it off. But before it runs away, the coyote snaps at the wing of the brave protector and injures it.

The juvenile bird is safe but the adult protector is not. Suddenly, the protector bird dies and begins to disintegrate. After a few minutes, another larger, stronger, and wiser bird appears. The protector bird is a phoenix.

As humans, we have the opportunity to rise anew as a phoenix in every opportunity where we squash our egos for the betterment of others. We should not consider it a diminishment of ourselves but a "rebirth." With each such rebirth in our lives, we move more steadily toward the realization of enlightenment.

We're not the most enlightened roles models we have Shakyamuni Buddha, Jesus Christ, Mohammed, Gandhi, Mother Theresa, and many others, filled with compassion for others? Didn't they put the needs of others before their own? This is what we need to do too. When it is in the higher good of all—be a phoenix!

On Wealth, Fame, and the Pursuit of a Really Great Loaf of Bread

The endless pursuit of wealth, power, and fame is highly over rated by most people. It is what drives some people to work excessively long hours, climbing their way to the top on the backs of others. Ultimately, this pursuit provides only an unhappy shell of existence.

To some, the attainment of wealth, power, and fame is at the core of their existence. The problem is that these states are not 100 percent compatible with being content. By their very nature, wealth, power, and fame are addictive. They have the hallmark qualities of addiction. No level is ever high enough. If other people get in the way, they may be crushed or hurt, and the drive to succeed replaces all other emotions. The life of the person addicted to the trappings of success eventually loses all joy.

The reality is that in life, you only are racing against yourself. Comparing yourself to others is useless and counterproductive. We never know the ultimate goal of a particular behavior of another person. We may believe that a person is doing action "A" to be successful because that is our goal and surely others would ultimately have the same goal as ourselves. However, the goal of the other person may be to maintain their sanity and get by with the least effort. So if we copy their behavior, then our behavior becomes counter-productive to our own goals.

Instead, if we develop personal goals of BEING and embodying compassionate wisdom, then our outlook on life and behaviors will be quite different. If we strive toward turning our lives into a really great loaf of bread, then the true riches of life, happiness, and contentment will follow.

Exercise: Great Bread Recipe

Ingredients:
- Understanding
- Patience

- Generosity
- Regular practice of caring and honest personal reflection
- Regular practice of chanting and meditation
- Better understanding of the pure universal teachings of spiritual co-existence among all people
- Compassion for all sentient beings—including oneself.

Directions:
Add all ingredients to your life. Gently knead and blend them into a consistent form. Smooth out all lumps. Let the dough sit and rise in a calm environment. Once raised to full height, bake in the glow of acceptance until content. Share with all you meet.

The Price is Right

Everything has a price associated with it. It could be the actual specific sales price or something of barter value if you traded for it. It could also have the value of the time that was required to obtain it. All of these are material payments and most likely not of extreme importance. The spiritual price one pays to hold onto an idea or "truth" is very different—it could be invaluable and might cost you your life.

Ideology has the power to make us royalty or paupers. Hitler used the ideology of the supremacy of an Aryan race to change the world forever. The Apartheid ideology was equally as powerful and damaging. Today, most people agree that these ideologies are wrong at any price, so it is no longer politically correct to hold these ideas.

However, there is a philosophy that is even more costly in terms of human lives that still goes unchecked today. In fact, it is such a strongly held belief by a huge percentage of the world's population that it is unhealthy for the planet, even the universe at large. This philosophy has already been mentioned in this text as a problem producer, but it bears mentioning again in a slightly different context. This philosophy states there is only one true religion and all other religions are dangerous.

To be saved for eternity, a person must ascribe to the one true religion philosophy whole heartedly. All other religions should be vanquished. The obvious problem with this idea is that the religion of "choice" is different around the world and across the street, sometimes even in the hearts of those that live under the same roof. So many lives have been sacrificed over the millennia to hold fast to this belief that they are impossible to count. It is time to stop the madness.

This is not a new observation—much has been written by scholars and activists about this terrible curse of inaccurate vision, but nothing has changed. A cursory internet search on the similarities of religions produces more sites about the differences than the similarities; however, there are some blogs and academic sites dedicated to spreading the understanding of the similarities. Some commonalities are the central theme of ethics, use of sacred art or imagery, sacred texts, concepts of powerful influences outside ourselves, and the belief that faith will change the lives of the adherents. Other sites list the "Ten Commandments" in various forms adopted by the different religions. All this is fine to point out, but really, it is made to be too complex.

The one simple similarity that is most important, which could save the world from self-destruction, is "compassionate wisdom." Pure and simple, it is making the best decision you can make with the intention of holding in mind the highest good for all sentient beings. Instead of the negative "Do no evil," adopt "Do only good with compassion in your heart for all." When this positive statement is adhered to in its purest form, all wars will stop, all abuse of every type will stop. All pain inflicted by man on man and animals will stop.

This is not a new concept—it has been understood for decades; so why has the population of the world failed to adopt it? One reason: "EGO!" The human psyche likes to feel it is part of an exclusively chosen group. They are the select few of the earth who know the "real truth" and only they will be "saved." What they do not understand is that no one will be saved or liberated from suffering until every last soul or person is also liberated from suffering. Since we are all physically connected by microscopically minute particle webs that are invisible to the naked eye, if you hurt, I hurt. This connection has been scientifically supported by distinguished astral physicists.

We must accept this concept that even those we consider to be our mortal enemies are really just extensions of ourselves. That which we hate about them is no more than a mirror of our own flaws. When we accept this fact and correct those flaws in ourselves, then we can accept the flaws in others.

To be able to recognize the mirrored flaws, we must practice compassionate wisdom. Compassion is needed to hold dear our immortal connection with all sentient beings. Wisdom is needed to be able to determine what action is in the best interest of all.

When compassionate wisdom is practiced in earnest, the price paid for a peaceful co-existence and global happiness is just right—the price is the elimination of suffering. Are you willing to pay the price?

Stop Trying to Do Good

We often praise people who are philanthropists because they give away a small portion of their great wealth to some organizations so that they can build a building or a charity that carries their name. Why do people give large or small sums of money to charities? Sometimes it makes good business sense because they need a tax write-off. Sometimes, they just want to support an organization because of what it does. Maybe, they want to feel that they are a part of it through their donations. They become a "member," such as when you donate to a public broadcasting station.

There are other good acts that we do that do not involve money. We can help our elderly neighbors cut the grass, donate time at our churches, become scout leaders or coaches for our children's activities. Why do we do these things? We might do it because it makes us feel good. We might want to provide lasting memories of good times. Maybe, we do it because we believe it is what we should do, the "right" thing to do.

People doing small acts of kindness every day makes life easier for those around them. What if we decide that we no longer are going to put intent behind our good actions? What if we decide to stop doing good deeds because "we want to help" or to "earn good karma" or "to make others happy" or to put someone in our debt, what would happen? What if we did good deeds without even thinking about it at all—is this possible? This is the state of perfect donation—this is when we begin to live our lives as grace—not in grace or merit, but as grace. This is when we become the true role model to guide others. This is when we do it right.

To do actions large and small without having the best interests of others in mind or your own best interest, but to do them just because it is a natural action to do, without any thought at all—this is when we get it right. This takes focused practice in the beginning; however, the more frequently you do something for the higher good of others without any intent, the sooner it will become part of your cellular makeup.

It is an interesting paradox. The harder you try to be remembered for your generosity, the less likely it will happen. The less you focus on your motives and live a life of pure donation and service, without intent, the more likely you will be remembered by an exponential number of people you touch. So begin your practice today. Reach out and touch someone, help without ulterior motives of any kind, make it your nature.

Exercise: Good Deeds without Intent

This exercise is one of the more difficult ones to accomplish. You have to improve your attention to detail and improve your ability to see what is before you without judgment.

- Begin by taking a walk anywhere you will see other people. You can walk outside or maybe around your office building.

- Walk around for the first 5 minutes, watch people, and observe your environment. Note the thoughts that are going through your mind. Most likely, your thoughts will run something like this: that yard is a mess, why didn't he park closer to the curb, she is just sitting on the porch doing nothing again, why didn't he shovel the snow from the sidewalk—how rude.

- Next, go up to someone and ask if you can help him or her with whatever they are doing. If they say no, continue walking and offering assistance until someone takes you up on your offer.

- What thoughts went through your mind when your offer(s) were declined?

- What thoughts went through your mind when you were assisting and after the task was completed?

Part Two: Practices

- It is common to feel a sense of pride and satisfaction after helping someone who does not expect to be helped. Doing something for others makes us feel like we are the "good guys."

- Second walk: Now shift gears and pay attention to your surroundings without judgment. Example: In one yard the grass is short, in another, the grass is long. One home has fresh paint, another one has peeling paint. There are flowers in one yard and gravel in another. Notice what the example did not say. It did not say the grass needs cutting or the house needs painting. The word "needs" establishes a judgment. Every judgment implies a right or wrong, a better or worse condition.

- Notice what the people you see are doing; for example, raking leaves, washing a car, getting groceries out of a car, walking down a corridor, or typing on a computer. Try to avoid judgment thoughts like, he is struggling with the leaves, he needs more soap to wash the car, the groceries look heavy, I bet she is answering her personal mail instead of working.

- Once again, you will help someone, only this time, go ahead and pick up another rake or shovel and start helping. Instead of asking, "Can I help you?" say "Two of us working together can get this job done more quickly." (Do not select a task that will take you into the home of someone you do not know. Obviously, your actions could be interpreted wrong or put you into danger.)

- The intent this second time around is to not judge yourself by your actions. This means that you do not pat yourself on the back for being a good neighbor or for being helpful. Just do what needs to be done without assessing the need or whether you should help or not.

- What was the response from the person you helped?

- How did you feel after helping out without judgment?

Continue this practice of just doing what needs to be done without judgment for one week. Assess how you feel afterwards. If you make this a life-long practice, you will completely change how you view yourself and your level of connectedness in the world.

19 Acknowledging Love

Love is the last of the spiritual traits and the outer layer of the spiral because it bathes all of the other traits in life-affirming energy. There are many other names for love, a few are universal life force, energy, spirit, God's love, and Buddha-nature. Its presence in the body determines the status of life or death. The energy itself never dies, it just moves on to a different body.

Gift of Life

"Life is precious." Although that phrase is commonly heard, few people know its true meaning. Many assume it means that we must be careful with our lives and the lives of others because they can be so easily snuffed out. Another interpretation is that each person is unique and therefore we must be careful not to harm any life. These assumptions are true when we focus on the word "precious."

There is also another meaning when the focus is on the meaning of "life." Life is more than the energy running through the body, without which we would be dead. Life is how we interact with the world. It is how we see ourselves as an integral part (or not) of the world and all of humanity. Life is the membrane that exists between our living selves and our "other" living selves. "Life" is the karma that keeps us rooted in our rebirth.

What are we really saying here? Life is the energy that we put forth on a second-to-second basis that is either contributing or not contributing to the level of compassion and acceptance in the world. Each breath every person on the planet takes either moves the whole of humanity forward on the compassion/acceptance scale, slides us backwards, or holds us in its current place.

It is only through acts of kindness done for NO reason without the expectation of reward or gratitude that the spiritual psyche of the world heals.

Deliberate acts of kindness are typically done with the expectation of gaining some recognition or quid pro quo. For example, a wealthy individual or corporation donates large sums of money to build a community ball field or convention center. In exchange, that individual or corporation's name is plastered on the marquee so everyone knows how "generous" they are. This is NOT generosity; it is marketing—visibility designed to improve business. If the corporation was truly generous, the donation would be anonymous AND they would not use it as a tax write-off.

The "gift of life" is truly rare and precious precisely because the human species rarely does anything without an agenda. Dogs, on the other hand, are actually much better at this than humans. They have no agenda when they wag their tails in happiness to greet their friends and providers. It is with pure natural joy that the tail wags and they pant in happiness.

We need to take cues from our loving pets. Be a source of unqualified happiness in the world. Develop an automatic smile that is triggered upon seeing another person. You need not speak in words—speak in smiles.

If a person needs assistance or just someone to listen to them without judgment, be there for them with an open ear and heart and no agenda. Do not attempt to influence them. Simply provide a mirror and a sounding board so they can see and hear themselves. No one can "fix" the suffering of another, but we can reflect back to others what is being projected into the space around them. Allow that space to be pure and untainted by your own prejudices. Provide the soft warmth of compassionate safety just to "be" who they are with all their failings, flaws, successes, and insights. Offer a safe zone with no expectations of any payback or required gratitude.

Life is about being like a flexible blade of grass that moves in response to external forces. Like grass, we need to allow others to pass into our lives but stay firmly rooted in understanding that we are a simple force of nature. We should be supportive of everyone with whom we come in contact and recognize that all of us are ever growing and changing.

Don't give to receive, give to give because it is the natural thing to do. Begin your "precious life" this moment.

Part Two: Practices

Love: Conventional and Otherwise

There is a lot of angry talk today about who can be legally married. One side of the debate says marriage should only be between a man and a woman; the other side says that couples of the same sex should be allowed to proclaim their love for each other and reap the benefits of a legal marriage. The whole question is silly—but important.

The question is silly because the gender of our physical body is really unimportant—it is merely a protective vessel to house our non-gender-specific spirit. With each reincarnation of the spirit into different vessels, it is a crapshoot as to the gender we will be each time. Well, sort of a crapshoot—it is more like a karmic lesson. We adopt specific genders and are placed in culturally specific bodies and regions so that we learn specific lessons based on our past lives. This allows us to pay back karmic debt and learn lessons in the new physical life that we did not learn before. A strongly misogynous male may come back as a female in a culture where women are treated as property. This would not be by chance but to learn tolerance and acceptance for all life.

Therefore, the question of marriage between same sex couples verses opposite sex couples is moot. Our spirit makes us who we are. That spirit has no gender, it just is. The spirit goes by many names—soul, Buddha-nature, essence, central life force, etc.—but whatever name you give it, it is that which when it leaves the body, the vessel ceases to have life. Whether that vessel was male or female makes no difference, it still is dead.

There are enough real issues in the world today over which people are fighting and killing. Why should the most sacred and important action that we can engage in—the reason for our embodiment—loving and caring for others be a cause of hatred? Love should always be celebrated and encouraged, regardless of the gender of the current vessel. It is the love and compassion that makes the person, not the gender.

On June 26, 2015, the United States Supreme Court took the surprising and remarkable step of legalizing same-sex marriage in all 50 states. They were right to correct this long standing discrimination but I am sure that this action will be contested at the state level for many years to come.

Friendship Today

Real friendship is rare. We may say we have many "friends," people who have electronically indicated that they want to be a follower of our lives from a distance. The notion is that the number of people we have "following" us on Twitter, Facebook, and other social media, reflects our popularity and status, but this is not true friendship.

Friends are people with whom we spend face-to-face, heart-to-heart time. Friends are people for whom we are willing to subdue our own needs, wants, and desires to help them obtain theirs. Friends are people who stick with us and provide a sounding board when we are confused, angry, in sorrow, or pain. Friends do not judge us. Friends support us. Unfortunately, few of us have someone in our lives that meet all of these requirements. So the question is—why is that?

Have we become so caught up in our own small world that we can no longer reach out to others? Have we become a prisoner to this world we created and put ourselves at the dead center? Are we buried so deep in our self-centered lives that we can no longer reach the periphery where other hearts exist? Has the digital world become a wall that separates us? Has this wall reduced our conversations to "K" and "LOL" to the point that even the soul of our language has been removed?

How did we devolve into a society of "me"? How do we create a society of "we"? How do we become authentic souls again? How do we bridge the gap of fear, doubt, and mistrust of our fellow humans?

It will not be easy to bring true friendship into our lives. If you look at all of the mass murderers over past generations, the one thing they all had in common was a sense of isolation and aloneness; they were disconnected from others at a heart level.

We need to heal our society. The way to do this is through unfettered acts of kindness and compassion for our neighbors. We need to pay real attention to others—seeing them, not seeing through them. We need to put the needs of others before our own. We need to become comfortable with all human conditions and support each other through them rather than ignore them. We need to reach out to those who cannot reach out for themselves. We need to learn the basic skill of listening without judgment, only love.

It is only through a web of connected hearts and hands that we thrive and flourish. Virtual webs might offer the illusion of connection but they are no substitute for the real thing. Reach out today for your own well-being and that of others. For we have seen only too often what happens when individuals disconnect from the loving support of others and fall out of the web.

Be there for someone today and every day. How can you make a difference in your own life and that of others? With whom can you reconnect today?

Charity—the Gift of Love to Yourself

What is charity? The typical definition of charity is to give something to someone in need. There are organizations specifically designed to help alleviate social need and provide services such as free meals, free/reduced-cost housing, monetary support, medical care, etc. We also use the term "charitable" to describe someone who speaks kindly of another or does not criticize when others think criticism is due.

Charity means much more than these explanations. To perform acts of charity means to perform acts of love. You might not even know the person that you are helping; this is the highest form of love.

The definition "to give something to someone who needs help" is a better definition ONLY when the actions are done from the goodness of the heart and with no ulterior motive other than love. The song "Love Makes the World Go Round" has it right. When we are extending a hand to others, everyone wins. You NEVER reduce your own supply of love and merit by giving it away to help others—you only increase it.

If you are feeling lonely and unloved, the thing to do is to donate your time and effort to help another. This is a gift to yourself too because it opens your own heart. Even if at first you do not feel loving when you extend your hand, the more you do it, eventually it will change your heart. When this happens, merit is gained and shared with the one you helped. This means that some of your karmic debt is lifted—not only yours—but the person being helped as well.

On airplanes, the flight attendant says, "Put on your own oxygen mask before you help others." Doing acts of charity is the same. You have to have love in your heart before you can share it. Selfish attitudes and behaviors only serve to increase the suffering in the world—including yours.

We are in a period of a "dark age." Materialism and technology fool us into believing that we are thriving when, in fact, this is not true. Never before in the history of man have so many who have so much refused to share. Never before have so many NOT recognized the contributions of others to their wealth. Instead, there is a mindset that "I pulled myself up, so can you." This is ridiculous—no one can succeed without the kindness of others. It is delusional to think so. It is an egotistical lie that we tell ourselves to justify selfishness. Hoarding our resources gained through the assistance of others results in the accumulation of karmic debt and divides society.

One of the great tenets of Buddhism is that the sangha (community) should not be divided. No one should attempt to divide the sangha for his or her own gain.

Refusing to help others causes a divide in the sangha or community and the rich get richer and the poor get poorer materially. However, in realty the rich also get poorer spiritually. It is as if their oxygen supply is being depleted, they are dying a slow death and they don't even recognize it. In the United States, today's climate of selfishness and fear is the harshest it has been in centuries. It is spiraling further out of control in ways that will impact generations to come.

Now is the time to extend the hand of love. Now is the time to show love for yourself by loving others. Now is the time to reduce your karmic debt by helping others to improve their physical lives and reduce their physical suffering. The remarkable thing is that those who are suffering physically typically share more of their love, time, and energy with others than those who are not.

Now is the time to step outside your comfort zone, remove your blinders of selfishness, and give back to the masses that gave to you. No one becomes prosperous in isolation. It takes others to get you there.

Exercise: Who Helped You?

In each of the sections that follow, think about the different aspects of your life. Identify persons that provided guidance, inspiration, encouragement, material assistance, opportunity, or anything else that has helped to make your life easier and more satisfying. Also, identify anyone who may have showed you the "wrong" way to do something, which inspired you to behave differently. For example, a parent that was incapable of being supportive and as a result you understand the pain from the perception of the child. Consequently, you make sure that you are always supportive of your children.

Family roles—Identify people who showed you how to be a better person in each of the following roles. Describe an incident that illustrates their role in your growth. Also include any one who provided negative examples. Use additional paper to write your responses as needed.

Parents:

Siblings:

Your Children:

Your Grandchildren:

Grandparents and Extended family members:

Circle of friends—Who taught you how to be a good friend? Describe how those lessons occurred:

Teachers:

Mentors:

Some people "blame" others for their negative traits and behaviors. Other people believe that they alone are responsible for their successes. In reality, we are the sum total of all of our experiences and interactions with others. Be grateful for all those who contribute to you. Extend your hand, guidance, and compassion to others as others have done for you.

What will you do for someone else?

20 Spaces Between the Layers—Ego and Grace

Without the spaces between layers, the spiral would fall in on itself. The spaces between the four inner ego traits are composed of ego. The spaces between the layers of the three spiritual traits are composed of grace. The spaces represent our two bodies: the physical body is supported by ego, and the spiritual body is supported by grace.

Life is Like a Box of Chocolates

There is a famous line in the movie *Forest Gump*, when the Gump character played by Tom Hanks says, "Mama always said, life is like a box of chocolates. You never know what you're gonna get." The literal meaning is that you never know what kind of candy filling you are going to get. It might be cream, truffle, cherry, raspberry, coffee, or any number of other confectionary creations. You try to eat the ones you like first, but you have to guess at what's inside and sometimes you bite into one you do not like. The analogous meaning of the lesson is, you never know what life will bring you. You do the things you like to do first, but there will always be things that you do not like. That is part of life, just like the chocolates you do not like are part of the assortment in the box.

Let's take the analogy a bit further in relation to the spiral. We talked about the spaces of the spiral being either ego or grace. The inner human traits are bound by ego and the spiritual traits are supported by grace. The transition between the two is fluid and ever changing. So how is this like assorted chocolates? All of us have our favorite fillings that make us smile, perk up our taste buds, and give us a warm sense of satisfaction. We also have ones we do not like and eating those is a punishment not pleasure; however, the chocolate shell can be eaten off and the filling avoided.

The ego traits of fear, anger, prejudice, and separation are like the chocolate coating around the undesired filling that punishes; it is attractive, even addictive, but if you bite in too far, it is punishing. Whereas the chocolate around our favorite filling is also just as attractive and addictive, when we bite into it, the resulting explosion of pleasure in our mouth is quite rewarding.

When we bite into the belief that acceptance, compassion, and love are desirable, we then feel more satisfied with life. The more we eat and experience the wonderful centers of the spiritual traits, the easier our life becomes. The good feelings send feedback to our brains that tell us that this is what we should be doing. Therefore, the more we practice acceptance and compassion, the more addictive that lifestyle becomes.

So why then do we continue to eat the chocolates that we really do not like? Old habits are easy. We do get some surface pleasure from feeding our ego. We do get some shell of pleasure from believing we are better than other people, that we stand apart and above them. However, the myth falls apart upon deeper inspection, as we go into the center of the chocolate, we realize that the bitter taste is really not what we want.

Rather than just nibbling off the chocolate shell for small insignificant ego-based "pleasure," choose to do only those actions and have those attitudes, thoughts, and beliefs that are supported by grace and that give you real and lasting pleasure every time you take a bite.

Exercise: Chocolate Sensation

Purchase a small box of chocolates with an assortment of fillings. There are sugar-free chocolates for those watching their sugar intake. You will also need a glass of water and a bowl.

1. If you can identify the fillings in each piece, select two pieces that you like very much and two that you do not like at all. Place them in front of you and have a glass of water available to cleanse your palate between samples.

2. Close your eyes and relax into a meditation. Allow your mind to run through the typical thoughts of work, family, or anything else that typically distracts you, and then clear your mind.

3. Begin with a piece with a less preferred filling. Allow the candy to sit on your tongue, and experience the sensation and taste of the chocolate. As it is melting think about an incident when you considered yourself better than someone else or

a time when your ego took the lead in your actions. Review the details of the event in your mind.

4. Just before the chocolate shell melts away completely, bite down into the center of the filling. As the filling sits on your tongue and melts away, think about how your actions impacted the other person at the time and how they also affect you in the long run.

5. After the candy has melted away, take a drink of water. Allow the water to sit in your mouth for a moment and then swish it around. Swallow the water. How do you feel about the water removing the taste from your mouth?

6. Repeat the process now with your favorite filling. This time while the chocolate shell is melting, think about a situation in which you accepted someone for who they are—faults and all.

7. Just before the shell melts away, bite into the filling. Remember the warm feeling the acceptance gave you.

8. After the candy has melted away, take a drink of water. Allow the water to sit in your mouth for a moment and then swish it around. Swallow the water. How do you feel about the water removing the taste from your mouth?

9. This time, place the second piece of candy that you do not like on your tongue and allow it to melt. Think about a time when you were angry with someone. Review the details of the event in your mind.

10. Just before the chocolate shell melts away completely, bite down into the center of the filling. As the filling sits on your tongue and melts away, think about how your actions impacted the other person at the time and how they also affect you in the long run.

11. Take a drink of water to cleanse the taste from your mouth. Allow the water to sit in your mouth for a moment and then swish it around. How do you feel about the water removing the taste from your mouth? Spit the water into a bowl. Is there a different thought in your mind after spitting out the water than what you had when you swallowed it before?

12. This time, place the second piece of your favorite candy on your tongue and allow it to melt. Think about the last time you acted with great compassion for someone. Review the details of the event in your mind.

13. Just before the chocolate shell melts away completely, bite down into the center of the filling. As the filling sits on your tongue and melts away, think about how your

actions impacted the other person at the time and how they also affect you in the long run.

14. Take a drink of water to cleanse the taste from your mouth. Allow the water to sit in your mouth for a moment and then swish it around. How do you feel about the water removing the taste from your mouth? Spit the water into a bowl. Is there a different thought in your mind after spitting out the water than what you had when you swallowed it before?

15. Go back into your meditation. In a relaxed, non-judgmental state, reflect on how each of the four experiences compared. Reflect on how much of your life you spend demonstrating the ego traits versus time spent demonstrating the spiritual traits.

16. Decide for yourself if you want more of your favorite chocolate life-expanding energy.

21 The Core—Trust

Trust is at the core of the spiral and our lives. If we truly trust that we are capable of changing our lives then we can. If we trust that all obstacles in our path are learning experiences then we do learn. Trust is the engine that drives improvement in our lives; without it nothing changes.

Trusting Your Instincts

At one time or another, we have all been told to trust our instincts. Teachers tell their students this before exams and they add, "Don't second-guess yourself."

What does this mean and why is it good advice? Isn't it better to ponder a question instead of immediately answering it? No, it isn't—in most cases. When we respond to situations from "instinct," we respond from our natural spiritual essence that already has access to universal knowledge and compassionate wisdom. The response will be well-grounded and appropriate for the situation. It will be for the higher good of all who are involved.

Conversely, when we respond from habit, or based in previous behavioral patterns, we are coming from a place fraught with emotional overlay that blinds us to the reality of the situation, and the reality of those involved.

Human behavioral patterns are incorrectly labeled "instinct" because they are often based in the ancient "flight or fight" response. This is a physical response that originated from our early evolutionary period. When we look at the extreme violence and cruelty in every part of the world today, we see the effect of this animalistic response.

The change in the vibrational rate of the planet, as a result of constant planetary movement in the galaxy, has caused an unsettled feeling in our physical bodies. The vast majority of people do not understand why they feel unsettled but it triggers a sense of fear, a guardedness to protect who they think they are. They have joined other equally fearful minds in groups, bands, gangs, political parties, societies, etc., to "defend" their view of life and behavioral patterns. They have "circled the wagons" around themselves to fight off some yet undefined threat call "change." As a human species, we seem to be moving back into the dark ages instead of moving toward a stronger period of enlightenment.

The reality is, however, that your physical body is not your essence. If we are going to go back to our most foundational and original selves, then we must connect with the universal energy—that which defines us, that which caused us to be able to breathe, that which lives long after the body has decayed and been replaced. Every one of us is not just connected to this universal energy—that always has been and ever will be—but we are a part of it.

Visualize if you will, the moment of the big bang that started the physical development of the universe. There was one bundle of energy that exploded and threw its particles into the 10 directions. The particles were not cleanly separated, they remained connected through a thin line not unlike a complex web we call the internet. Every particle or "spirit" (for lack of a better word) is connected.

This vibrational energetic connection is who we are. We are the essence of the universe. Every one of us is connected and we are all the same, exploded out of the same source. Not as siblings, but as part of the whole and equal in every way because there is no distinction.

It is only the protective shell, our physical bodies, which we have adopted to function in this vibration plane that sees distinctions. These are false distinctions colored by fear, greed, desire, ego, and most critically, lack of true self-identity.

If we understand this and live our physical lives from our "true selves," there would be no wars, no terrorism, no bickering over what is mine and what is yours, no question of how the physical resources of the world should be divided and used. Like water, these resources would flow to the low spots from places of abundance and equalize out. The difference is a raging sea with high waves and deep valleys that can (and does) trigger devastation, versus a calm, flat, peaceful sea that invites all to fish and play together in the warmth of the sun.

Part Two: Practices

So, the next time you need to make a decision or respond to something—trust your true instinct. Don't just repeat dysfunctional human behavioral patterns. Use the network of compassionate intelligence that is heart-based, not fear-based and ego-driven. Don't second guess yourself into a lower-level solution.

Unfinished Objects (UFOs)

An UFO in the quilting world refers to an "unfinished object." It is a project or quilt that we began, gave energy to, but for one reason or another we put it down unfinished. Maybe the elements were not coming together as planned. Maybe we lost enthusiasm for it or maybe we were distracted by another idea that seemed to hold more promise. Maybe it proved to be too difficult and the quilter was not up to making the effort, to acquire the skills, to solve a problem, or they tried but the solution eluded them. Regardless of the reason, that bud of a project is put into a bag and placed in a drawer. Maybe the quilter will take it out periodically and look at it again—maybe not.

There are UFO swap groups where people exchange their UFOs to complete. The rules are, there are no rules. The new person can do whatever they feel drawn to do with the UFO within a specified period of time, and then return it to its owner with the problem solved their way.

This is a great metaphor for life. Sometimes we face a problem that we just do not know how to solve. We put it away from our consciousness by alcohol, work, material accumulation, power, or denial. We might occasionally bring it to our consciousness when we are feeling stronger, or it might bubble to the surface when we are quiet or trying to do something else. It is only when the problem really starts screaming from the depths of the shadows do we seek assistance in solving it.

If the quilter of life belonged to a guild—a community of quilters, a sangha—she or he could have brought up the project/problem in its early stages when things were not jelling. Guild members know that every one of them have UFOs somewhere in a drawer, so they are very willing to help. When one member asks for help and receives it with loving support, it then becomes much easier for other members to ask for help too. Bringing your issue to light is helpful because, most likely, others also have similar problems tucked away, unacknowledged, but unforgotten.

So get your guild members together; call your sangha to order, invite your family for a sit-down, or gather your friends together. Declare a UFO Day where everyone brings a problem to the table. Get fresh eyes on the situations and bring in other people's field of experience to solve the questions.

Exercise: UFO Day

1. Announce an "UFO Day" in advance. Tell members to come prepared with their UFO to hand off to someone else.

2. Give everyone a pad of paper and a pen. Spend about 10 minutes having everyone write about his or her UFO. DO NOT PUT NAMES ON THE PAPER TO IDENTIFY THE SOURCE.

3. Place all of the notepads in a pile and shuffle them, then distribute them back out to the group.

4. In round-robin-fashion, pass the notebook around. Each person in the group should write his or her solution on a separate page in the notebook from the question and previous answers. Each person should read what others have written and come up with something different and unique. You can also add to something someone else wrote on their page as long as it takes the solution a step farther. No criticism or negation is allowed!

5. When your own tablet comes to you, follow step 4 just as if it were someone else's, not your own.

6. Continue passing the tablets until everyone has written on all of the tables. If the group is large, break it up into smaller groups to finish in a timely manner.

7. Return the tablets to the original writers. Read the solutions.

8. Have a meditation session to allow the possible solutions to gel and have your spirit guides help you through it.

9. Warmly hug all of your supporters in gratitude.

10. Take the solutions home with you for reference and try them out.

The Glue that Holds Relationships Together—Trust

Children are so wonderful in their innocence. Young children have no sense of lying or mistrust. Young children believe the world centers around them; this is natural. Their brains have not yet developed enough to think otherwise, but even in their self-centeredness, they love unconditionally. They trust that others will have their interest at heart.

Older children and young adults lose this pure state. Oftentimes teenagers no longer trust their parents. Rather than loving everyone unconditionally, they form exclusive cliques.

Popular teens can be cruel to those who are not popular. The targets of distain develop scars that carry over into adulthood if left unchecked.

The shift from giving and receiving unconditional love to being the target of cruel barbs and pranks can (and does) do emotional harm and sets back the development of healthy relationships. If teens are not able to form friendships with any of their peers, real damage can occur. They may lose their innate ability to trust. We must trust that there is a place for us in society. We must trust that we are equal to and part of the whole of humanity. We have to find our place. If as a young adult, we do not find a safe and accepting place, normal development into adulthood is delayed.

It is interesting that we can continue to love someone who hurts us, but once we lose our trust in that person, it is very difficult to reestablish it. Once the trust is broken, the relationship often fails shortly thereafter. Trust is the glue that holds relationships together. Trust is what holds families together.

Trust in yourself is just as important as trust in others. If we lose trust in our ability to make good decisions for ourselves, we can become paralyzed in our ability to function. We are more likely to turn control of our lives over to someone else, and that puts us in danger of giving control to a person who may have only his or her own self-interest in mind.

What then do we need to do to protect ourselves? We need to assess our trust in ourselves and in others. We need to repair the important relationships with our families and with ourselves.

Exercise: Trust

1. Critically assess how you view your decision-making abilities. Do you believe that you are capable of making the right decisions for yourself, even if you have not done so in the past?

If the answer is no, analyze the last several decisions you made that you consider to be faulty. How did you arrive at the decision? What could you have done better?

Part Two: Practices

Do you see a pattern in how you arrived at the poor decisions? If so, what is the pattern?

2. Devise a plan, a standardized procedure for your personal decision-making process in the future. If you cannot trust yourself, trusting others will be very difficult.

Part Two: Practices

3. You have already analyzed your most difficult relationships in the exercise "Assess Your Relationships." Go back and reread what you wrote.

   What was your role in breaking the trust between you and the other people? If you believe that it is entirely the other person's fault, you are probably in denial. Dig deeper to discover your role.

4. Ask to have a real conversation with the other person. Apologize for your role in the problem. Even if the other person does not apologize, it is essential for you to claim your contribution. It is impossible for us to grow if we do not acknowledge our mistakes. Write the script for what you will say. It is better to think this through in advance rather than "wing it." If you script what you need to say, you are much less likely to go on the defensive and fall back into old patterns of blame and denial.

5. Forgive yourself and forgive the other person. Repeat the exercise "Forgiving to Eliminate Suffering," in Forgiveness Part III (page 36). When you begin to rebuild trust in yourself, the ability to trust in others will follow.

Part Two: Practices

Part Three: Additional Practices

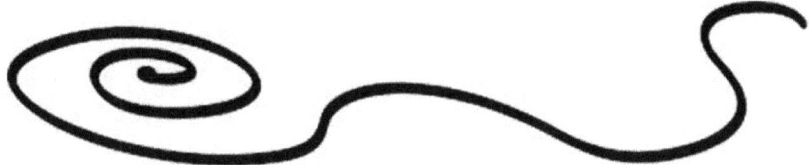

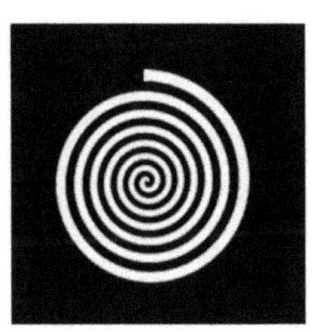

Part Three: Additional Practices

Reflective Readings to Illustrate Other Critical Practices

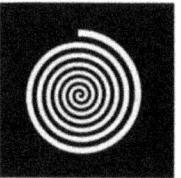

This section introduces practices for additional behavioral changes that support and enhance the foundational practices of the spiral.

22 Attachment

Attachment refers to our inability to let go of things, ideas, and control of others and our environment. We tend to hold onto things out of habit or fear because we identify with it even though it may no longer really represent our current thinking and beliefs. We hold onto false ideas of what we are capable of accomplishing. The attachment to the idea of inadequacy is a self-fulfilling prophesy. We hold attachments to more negative and self-defeating ideas than positive ones. When we let go, a whole new world of possibility opens up to us.

Forgotten Existence

Is it possible to forget who we are? People who have suffered a severe head injury sometimes have amnesia and cannot remember who they are. What about those who have not suffered an injury, can they forget?

Sadly, many people in life do not remember who they are. They may identify themselves by their life roles, their job, or the identity that someone else gave them instead of their essence.

What is our essence? It is the breath that sustains us, without which we would be no more. Our personal history—our stories are important to our ego-centered nature but what if we could not remember our stories? What if our slate for this lifetime was wiped clean? What if we could begin from scratch, re-creating ourselves without karmic payback to complete? What would we do?

Essentially, this is possible with each passing moment. Since each moment is new, yet-to-be-written, we have the opportunity to construct it the way we wish. Maybe you cannot change your physical surroundings if, for example, you are in prison. But you can determine where your emotions, mind, and thoughts will be, and this directly controls your situation.

If you want your true essence to shine through, you will need to consciously set aside the exact emotions, thoughts, and experiences to which you so dearly cling. Don't let the past "old news" define your present. Instead, let your essence shine through to define you.

Begin by thinking with your heart. This is not to say you should let your emotions rule you—absolutely not. By using the tools of the Eightfold Path and the Six Perfections, combined with a loving heart, we will always know what to do. (These Buddhist tools are explained in the glossary along with how to use them.)

Crying

Crying is underrated as an emotional behavior. Some men refuse to do it. In many cultures, young boys are taught not to do it. "Big Boys Don't Cry" is not just the name of a song. This is unfortunate because the act of crying—shedding water in the form of tears—is very cleansing.

The release of pent up emotions allows the body to rebalance. Yes, it is exhausting and afterwards you may feel as though you were run over by a train, but it is the body's way to relieve anger, frustration, or pain as a safe nonviolent response. Tears use the body's natural water content to wash away the emotional build up, but it does come with that run-over-by-a-train feeling.

Mindful release, on the other hand, works just as well, but without the train factor. By visualizing the release of your pain or suffering, and then actually letting go of it, your body will feel relief and freedom, instead of feeling squashed.

The problem with this is that many people will not let go of their pain even though they claim they want relief from it. Pain becomes a self-identifier, it is familiar, and it is predictable. If "A" happens, then I will feel the painful but predicable "B." If I drink too much, I will have a head-splitting hangover in the morning. No one likes change, even if it might make us feel better.

If we give ourselves permission to wallow in the painful emotion for only a limited time, feel the experience in every fiber of our being, allow it to well up, and then consciously shed it, the ensuing relief will be healing.

Consider the pressure cooker; with the lid off, the boiling water will eventually fully evaporate. It will take awhile, but eventually it is spent. With the lid on, with no pressure release (i.e., no crying), then eventually when a tiny crack appears in the seal, an explosion will occur. If you vent the pressure cooker, the steam will quickly escape and the volume of water remains about the same; it is not completely spent—so it is with mindful release.

Part Three: Additional Practices

Exercise: Getting Control of Your Pain

Determine the category of the source of your pain and visualize that you are coloring it a specific color based on its source chakra. (See the glossary for more information on chakras.)

- Red (pubic region)—basic material issues

- Orange (just below the navel)—relationships, creativity blocks

- Yellow (just above the navel)—low self-esteem, feeling unworthy

- Green (heart)—loss of a loved one through death, divorce, or separation

- Blue (base of the throat)—anger at ourselves for not being able to speak out against injustices done to our loved ones or ourselves, communication problems in general

- Indigo (third eye)—feeling the pain of separation with our spiritual self

- Crown (top of the head)—connection point with the universal life energy

The primary channel for energy to travel through our body is through the spinal column. There are many, many smaller chakra points in the body but only seven primary ones as noted above.

1. To open your chakras, visualize opening the crown chakra and bringing in the white shimmering light of the universe and running it down your spine.

2. Visualize each opening of your body based upon the locations listed above. Then visualize a funnel of colored light about 18 inches in diameter spinning clockwise out of the front of the port and the same funnel of light spinning counter-clockwise out of the back from your spine at the same point. Each funnel should be of the same diameter and spinning at the same velocity. Opening each of your chakras allows you to use them as emotional vents.

3. Once you have established open funnels of the appropriate colors, visualize your pain the same color as the corresponding chakra, again based on the information above. Once you have colored it, visualize spinning the pain right out of your body.

Example: To release pain resulting from security needs or lack of material support. Visualize red base chakra (in the pubic region) opening and red gas of suffering escaping.

By visualizing the pain as a color, you neutralize it and it goes into the environment purified. Changing the pain into a color and releasing it also empowers you to gain control of the emotions that once controlled you. What is left afterward is a sense of weightlessness, lighter, and freer. The steam of suffering will be released.

The process of classifying the source helps you to understand its control over you. Coloring and releasing the pain helps you to regain control in a loving way. No train wreck feeling afterward—just relief. While a good cry is temporarily cleansing, mindful release is healing.

Asleep Standing

Sometimes when we are feeling exhausted, we might find that there are periods when we lose memory of events. For example, we drive home but upon arriving, we do not remember the actual drive. We put our bodies on automatic pilot while we do mundane tasks. We walk through our day asleep, in a fog—day after day after day.

Sometimes the memory lapses or fog can be blamed on sleep deprivation, but the most likely reason is deprivation of purpose, for when we are living "in purpose" we are awake! Awake to the task at hand, awake to the meaning of our actions, awake to the thoughts in our minds. When we live with purpose, it becomes easier to see the true reality of our experiences without the shroud of ego coloring it. We are less likely to set up a confrontational situation because of misreading the situation.

When we live each moment with purpose, instead of pushing for a future goal or reliving past experiences, we are more effective. When we block out sabotaging self-chatter that reduces our self-worth, we become free to be, free to do what is called for at the precise moment it's needed. It is only by living with the single purpose of focusing on this very moment that we succeed in moving along on our path to becoming awake.

We are awake when we live each moment easily without intent, without forcing thoughts or actions—just being awake and seeing what the true nature of our existence is at every moment. We are awake when we do not judge the situation—we just live it. We are awake when we live in full gratitude for each moment regardless of the events that are occurring.

To be awake is our natural state of being. Our ego-self is the culprit that tries to obscure the truth from view—the connectiveness of all things and all people. When we see the world through the eyes of our egos, we see a very different place. No longer do we see in gratitude, but instead the world is veiled in entitlement. This sets us up for disappointment and suffering that is self-inflicted. It doesn't have to be so.

If you want to change your life, it is within your power to do so. In fact, only you have this power—no one else can change you. When you change your perspective and see the moment through eyes of gratitude, things become clearer. You are more likely to see the true reality of the events unfolding.

When we see through eyes of entitlement, clarity will always be displaced by delusions. Therefore, if you want to live with less suffering—it is simple. Change how you see—change your perspective. Do what comes naturally and just be—be in each moment with gratitude.

Changing Old Floor Covering

When you own a home, every so often you need to make major repairs. The roof needs to be replaced, paint needs to be updated, and floor coverings needs to be replaced. It's expensive to make these repairs. To replace the flooring covering, it takes not only lots of money, but also lots of time. Typically, we will peel back the old carpet or linoleum and see how the wood foundation looks. All of the broken boards need to be repaired before new covering can be put into place. The furniture needs to be moved to another room, flooring changed, and then the furniture is moved back.

Periodically, we also need to assess ourselves. What habits and thoughts do we have that are old and out of date; what no longer serves our needs? We need to peel back these old habits and see how our foundational core looks. Is it in need of repair? How has it changed? Does it need upgrading too?

Updating and fixing ourselves is infinitely more costly and difficult than changing the floor covering. The cost is in having to admit that what we are currently doing is not working. The image we are presenting to the outside world is not who we really are. We may even have to admit we are wrong about some of our long-held beliefs. Maybe the environment in which we live has changed so significantly that our beliefs are no longer valid.

Letting go of old beliefs and habits is extremely difficult because, over time, we begin to believe that we are what we think and do. We view ourselves as liberals or conservatives, traditional or new age, daring or risk adverse, introverted or extraverted, happy or depressed, creative or uncreative, and on and on. These labels define us in our own minds and to the outside world but they are not who we really are and certainly they are not fixed and unchanging over our lifetime. We change, and others change too.

To change, we need to go through the letting go process. We need to break the mythical linkage between what we think and who we think we are. We need to conduct a serious search of our soul, our spiritual essence to understand what our spirit is seeking for nourishment. Sometimes this period is called a "middle-age crisis" but it can happen at any age and occurs more than just once in our lifetime. We can ignore our spiritual needs and immerse ourselves in the material world for only so long. Eventually our spirit cries out to us like a squeaky floorboard, "Pay attention to me!"

How do we fix our spirit? How do we renew our soul? How do we select new covering? How do we know that the covering we select at the store will be suitable? Can we return our selection if it is not right for us? These are all questions that, if unanswered, may prevent us from taking the leap to change. Let's address each one.

How do we fix our spirit? The process is deep reflection and assessment of what is working in our lives and what is not working. We need to look at what brings us peace and contentment and what causes pain in our lives or to others. Reflect on the following questions:

- What are you doing that is causing pain to the people who are closest to you?
- Are you angry?
- Do you say things, knowing that the words will push buttons and cause pain?
- Do you act out by throwing things or giving the silent treatment, causing the entire household to suffer?
- Do you lie about what you are really feeling because you feel it is safer and easier than telling the truth?
- Do you go places without your spouse that might tempt you to cross a line that you know you should not cross?
- Do you think less of others and allow a false sense of superiority to prevent you from interacting and understanding others on an honest plane?
- Do you think about the repercussions before you speak or act?
- Do you consider others as important as yourself and therefore deserving of your time, attention, and consideration?

There are an infinite number of questions that could be asked to assess our current standing. The important thing is that we are open to an honest look at our beliefs, attitudes, and behaviors. Are we adding to the light of the world or are we a black hole, sucking the life and energy out of our relationships?

How do we renew our soul? We quiet our minds and still our bodies. A cleanse is needed after our period of reflection. Find a tree in a quiet location. Place your spine against the tree and relax. Clear your mind of worries, focus on your breathing, allow the fresh air to fill your lungs, and relax. If the weather is such that an outdoor cleanse is not possible, find an indoor space that is peaceful, free of emotional associations, and has soothing energy.

How do we select new covering? Reflection by itself is somewhat worthless; correction is required to make the change. The one thing we do not want to do is to go into the abyss of guilt. Feeling guilty only serves to prevent us from thinking clearly. It is like a wet towel thrown over us, preventing us from moving freely, preventing us from changing. Guilt is never helpful. This is not the same as admitting we were wrong or admitting that we should have done something different. The emotional baggage of guilt is like a chain that is difficult to break. Honest reflection of our own role in producing our current emotional pain is essential to eliminating it. Apologizing for our errors actually breaks chains of guilt. When we take responsibility for creating our suffering, we are in control of creating our peace. We select the new covering by determining what would bring us inner peace.

How do we know that the covering we select at the store will be suitable? The "store" refers to the cornucopia of beliefs and behaviors available to us. Let's go back to the floor covering analogy—we may select a carpet that does not coordinate with the curtains, sofa, cabinets, or chairs. The question becomes then, are these other "furnishings" also in need of change? Do your current attitudes, beliefs, and behaviors suit your needs well or are they part of the problem? If they are part of the problem, then they also need to be replaced. Keep them if they are working in your life. We can tell they are working if they bring us peace and also bring peace to others that are sharing the space. It is extremely important that those with whom we live also be at peace. Fixing one squeaky floorboard but not another leaves the problem unsolved.

One trap to be aware of is that we all have favorite colors and shapes to which we are attracted and tend to repeat in our surroundings and clothes. Are these really in your best interest? This is not a time to fall back on what is comfortable. Be bold, be brave, select what will move you further on your quest for happiness—your quest for self-improvement—your quest for establishing a peaceful environment around you.

Can we return our selection if it is not right for us? Yes. The beauty of life is that we can and do change on a daily basis. Once we have decided to chart a new course free of our former attachments, changing beliefs and behaviors becomes easier. It's extremely freeing to realize that if we have no attachment to what we think is right, we are free to accept what is right for each individual scenario in which we might find ourselves.

It is infinitely rewarding to take the time to answer all these questions. Once you do, you can take the leap to change. You will be happy you did.

23 Peace

Peace is one of those things that everyone says that they want but no one knows how to obtain. Peace and attachment go hand-in-hand. When we give up the craving to control and acquire then we have an opportunity to be at peace within ourselves and with others.

What is Peace?

Peace is much more than simply an absence of war between nations. It is more than not fighting with your neighbor. Peace really begins with you not fighting with yourself. When you are at total peace with who you are, what you are capable of, where you are going in life, what you have and do not have, then you will be at peace.

It's not possible to promote peace honestly among others when there is no peace within yourself. If we have never felt peace within ourselves, then we have no frame of reference for how it feels, what it looks like, or how it tastes or sounds. We have no notion of how to obtain it or recognize it when it exists. Therefore, we must cultivate peace within ourselves first.

The number one obstacle to peace is desire: desire for power, desire for material and financial gain, desire for recognition. Desire for whatever one feels would give him or her an edge to stand above and over others. This is not peace—it is tyranny. A person who has these desires will surely abuse anyone who stands in their path to attain them.

Peace and power really are the same thing but not in the usual sense of the meaning. Power is required to have peace. You must have the power to control your own desires and your own greed. Once you have established complete control over your basic animal urges, then peace will find its way in—not until then.

Accumulated material wealth demands more power over others and demands increasing amounts of power to maintain control. Lies take more lies, to maintain secrecy. So if you want peace—STOP. Stop your cravings and desire for things that do not build peace of mind, peace of spirit, peace of soul, or peace of your essence. Root out the cause—desire. Clear the black shroud of greed from your being. Be satisfied with what you have and do not have. Better yet—give away much of what you have—you really do not need it anyway. Once shed of desire and material weight, then and only then is there room for peace to come in. If there is no space available, how will peace be able to take root and grow? Make space, and then share.

Part Three: Additional Practices

Wanting Peace and Getting It

What does it mean when one says that he or she wants peace? Peace is a fairly elusive concept. Peace is timely as we have frequently witnessed. Peace can be between nations or communities. It can also be between individuals of warring nations while their respective military and politicians continue to rain down their bombs and bullets.

Does peace between individuals need to be a Shakespearian tragedy? No, it does not. What must happen for peace to occur and war to stop?

Each winter holiday season, we hear the song *Peace on Earth, Goodwill Toward Men*. It can be heard playing daily on our radios, in stores, and restaurants. People sing about it in their homes but rarely are the messages expressed from the heart.

A review of American history since 1776 shows that our country has been engaged in war for about 90 percent of the time since we have been a nation. One war (or conflict) may end while another one is brewing on the horizon. How many more lives must be sacrificed in the name of justice, democracy, religion, retaliation, revenge, self-rule, or freedom from tyranny?

It begins on the personal level—letting go of hate and revenge, seeing others as one with ourselves, appreciating the similarities instead of focusing on the differences. Take the time to get to know your neighbors, practitioners of other faiths, and people of other nationalities. Become enriched by these friendships instead of afraid of the differences.

Are you up to the challenge to do your part?

24 Healthy Behaviors

There are other healthy behaviors that lead to a life filled with joy and reduced suffering. Here are stories that point the way.

The Center of All Life

Life begins with thought, a breath, and a signal of life. The breath is a whisper from the universe that all are connected and good. There is no matter too small or large that does not hold life's compassionate energy. All in the universe thinks its own way. A rock does not worry about what it will wear to dinner that night but instead its consciousness is focused on just being. A tree is focused on just being. As humans, we clutter our most precious and gifted minds with useless thoughts. We create pain for ourselves stemming from desire and a sense of lacking that is artificial and of no use to the universe.

Part Three: Additional Practices

If we could follow the example of the rocks and earth and just BE, our ability to experience fully our role in the web of life would be limitless. It is only through BEING that we can have a fundamental base that lovingly serves all sentient beings in this universe.

The ripple effect of pure being, unencumbered by judgment and desire, heals all. The web is strengthened through nonjudgmental being, but clogs up with anger, fear, separation, and prejudice.

The web cannot be broken, but when it's in a clogged state, acceptance, compassion, and love have a more difficult time flowing. The following three attitudes/actions are the essence of all life—of all sentient beings:

1. Acceptance that all is as it should be. All is where and what it needs to be, at that time, and in that place.

2. Compassion for oneself as part of the web of life, seen with a clear heart that guides all actions.

3. Love, in its purest form, is the basis of the foundation. It is the motor for acceptance and compassion. It is the organic, life-sustaining substance, like water for a flower, without which all will wither.

Pure unconditional love is practiced on a nanosecond-by-nanosecond basis by all beings except humans. These three attitudes/actions form the structure of the web that supports human life. They encourage human life to become one with them in an open, flowing network of compassionate energy that feeds and nurtures all.

It is only the human link in the chain that self-destructs and sabotages itself and others (both other humans and non-humans.)We have the ability, more than other sentient beings, to strengthen and clear the clogged arteries of the universal web. Up to now, most people have chosen to dedicate their lives to acquiring things. "The one who has the most toys wins." Nothing could be further from the truth. It is only through shedding the trappings of desire and accumulation that BEING can possibly take place.

The human world must get back to the basis of being to become healthy again. The health of the universe depends on humans to do their part to open up their clogged arteries and renew the health of the whole web.

Without this conscious, mindful effort at reestablishing acceptance, compassion, and love to BE again, the human link will continue to weaken the health of the entire network.

Make the conscious effort NOW and every moment to be present in all you do, to accept all things and every person on their own terms, without judgment. Sow the seeds of compassion in your everyday thought and action. Water the entire web with love, starting with yourself. The only sentient beings that do not love themselves and recognize their own self-worth are humans. The evolution of sophisticated digital communication has weakened our ability to communicate with a clear mind and heart. We must regain what we have lost and put acceptance, compassion, and love back into a practice of BEING.

Exercise: Practice of Being

Be still for a moment. Eyes can be opened or closed.

- Breathe into your heart acceptance for who you are. Allow acceptance to flood every cell of your being. Feel it radiate out and bring alive all of your senses.

- Breathe in compassion into your heart. Feel its warmth flood over you. Feel its texture and substance. Savor the sensation for a couple of minutes.

- Finally, breathe love in through your heart, all the love to cement acceptance and compassion within you. Now see how different it feels from the other two. Feel its grounding sensations as you breathe it in deeply.

- Rest for a few moments and be at one with the sensations. Accept this knowledge, feeling, and force as you—just BE. Repeat this exercise throughout the day, especially when you feel stressed. Just BE and enjoy it.

Where Did the Wild Ones Go?

Once we are past our early thirties, our everyday existence could feel as though it has become hum-drum and boring. Maybe on a weekend we might have an evening of pleasant discussion or see a movie, but life would not be labeled wild and crazy.

What is it that causes us to change from a fun-loving teen to a sedate mature person? Where does our spontaneity go?

One theory is that we squash our enthusiasm for life because we learn as a child (under the age of 7) that we are rewarded when we "behave," and showing wild enthusiasm is "misbehaving." Therefore, by the age of 21 we have learned to sedate the life out of ourselves for public approval.

This approach could not be further from the truth. Learned self-control is not equal to killing off your emotional energy bodies. Allowing your emotions to whip you around from high to low and all about is not a desired state, it only makes one dizzy.

When we are mindful and in the moment, we do feel the joy of life. We understand what is going on with complete clarity, without the blinders of living in past guilt, or in the rose-colored future to distort our impressions. The sensation we feel is like a warm, soft, encompassing glow, which brings a smile to our faces and a sense of contentment settles over us. Why go jumping around like a firecracker when being still brings such pleasure? It is impossible to have clarity of mind if you are jumping about, and impossible not to have clarity if you are still in your being. Maturing is not about denying oneself the pleasures of a wild life; it is about learning how to be in tune with your life.

To feel this intense pleasure, you must be willing to open the door to it. This is done by spending time each day just "being" in quiet reflection or meditation. Meditation is better than reflection; in reflection we tend to beat up on ourselves for every little thing we perceive we have done wrong.

Instead, quiet your mind; be fully aware of your surroundings, yet not absorbed into it. Quiet your body and mind for a period of time each day to allow your senses to recharge and bounce back from the barrage of stimuli that is showered in on a minute-by-minute basis. No wonder adults feel they must be sedated. They must shield themselves from the constant bombardment of stimuli, that comes with multi-tasking and living an electronic existence. Humans have become like robots, programmed to patch into the command center—smart phones, computers, music devices—to receive their direction for life or to provide distraction, so that they don't have to experience the moment.

Hand-held portable devices have been hailed as the technology that has improved lives and connected people. Instead, the reality is that they have done just the opposite. People rarely make eye contact as they walk down a street or sit in a room full of people, because they are tuned into their own little shuttered headphone world.

How can you be open to the possibilities of a moment-to-moment awareness when you are deaf to your environment? So improve your life—unplug—turn off the electronics, experience a renewed relationship with your environment and those in it.

Embrace the duality—stimulation and calm—that comes from being fully present in your everyday life. You will be amazed how it will feel. The pleasure days of your wild youth will return, but in a way that is calmer, steadier, and provides you with clarity instead of a hangover.

Free Will

We believe that we have free will to choose to do what we want to do when we want to do it. We believe that ultimately every behavior is a result of a conscious decision. On the surface, this is correct. You can choose to eat peanut butter or cheese. You can choose to meditate daily or not. But if you have a peanut allergy or are lactose-intolerant, the food selection is somewhat less free. If you have not planned your schedule to wake up early before going to work, this also becomes a less free choice of what you eat for breakfast. Clearly, we have more control over our sleep/wake schedules than our food allergies—or do we?

The law of cause and effect is at the root of all decisions and behaviors; for example, a person who feels as though his spouse or partner is ignoring him may "accidentally" eat something that triggers a physical illness. The partner will then feel sympathy and become more attentive. The first couple of times, the spouse's response will be genuine concern, but if the behavior continues, the spouse may become annoyed because the loved one brought the illness on himself. However, even the spouse's show of annoyance is a form of attention. Negative attention is still attention and it's better than being ignored.

Clearly, eating something that we know will make us sick is not in our highest interest. So why do it? Why not find another way to satisfy the need for attention? Why not eliminate the need for attention entirely? Is this even possible? Is this desirable? If a person is able to be content with his or herself, if they have successfully squelched their greedy craving for attention, then they change their choice of behavior changes. Better decisions regarding what is in our higher good can be made.

The cycle of cause and effect is still at play but the desire to improve your walk on the path in life changes. Different forks in the road are taken. Both forks will ultimately provide a learning situation, the exact one you need at that time. You will either be presented with a repeat scenario of something you should have learned from a previous experience but did not, or you will be presented with a new scenario that will help you to understand something different about yourself.

Ultimately, every choice we make in life teaches us something. How often we are presented with the same learning experience dressed in slightly different clothing is entirely up to us. We do have free will to make decisions but those situations in which we must decide are preset. They are preset by our previous decisions to learn or not learn.

Your ability to live the life you want is entirely predicated on whether or not the life you want is in your highest good. We may want to be powerful, to have the full attention of others, or to have unlimited financial resources, but ultimately none of these will move us further toward our spiritual goal of enlightenment.

Until we align our earthly goals with our spiritual goals, we will be presented with challenges that will help us learn to make the right choices toward our full development. We cannot escape the effect of our choices. So instead of repeating the same dukka (suffering), always make the choice to consider what is in your own highest good. Take the wiser fork in the road instead of the easiest one.

Healthy Living

Each new year, vast numbers of people make New Year's resolutions to live a healthier life style. They vow to lose weight by eating better and exercising more. Typically this resolve lasts three to maybe five weeks (or days) and they are back to their old habits. Then they feel like a failure in addition to feeling unattractive—a double whammy. The key to living a healthy life lies not in what we put in our mouths, but what we put in our hearts.

The second key is exercise. Lift karmic weights as a life practice, not just metal ones in a gym. Start by finding a personal trainer that is skilled in spiritual arts; someone who understands how to use the proper spiritual exercise machines. Effective ones are the Four Noble Truths, The Eightfold Path, and The Six Perfections (see the Glossary). There is another machine called the Ten Commandments, from the Bible, that if you use positive movements instead of negative, it works well too. By doing these exercises you will begin to get your heart in good condition, your mindset will change, and you will be more disposed to feed yourself correctly.

So, of what should your heart-healthy diet consist? Instead of the pyramid of food groups, we should be following the plate model because it better represents the perfect balance of foods that provide a well-rounded diet.

The first food group is acceptance. This is acceptance that everything in your life is just as it should be for you to learn the lessons you need to lift those karmic weights. Acceptance that you are connected to everyone in the "gym" and we need to be spotting each other, so that if one of those weights begin to fall too heavily on others, we can assist them in stabilizing the load until they can rest a moment and regain their strength and confidence to continue working toward their goals.

The second food group is compassion. Compassion is a vitamin, and has no fat. The best quality of this food group is that it feels good going down. It also has a cleansing effect on our systems and bodily organs. It removes the lodged impurities that get stuck on a cellular level and flushes them clean. The guilt, self-loathing, separateness, and lacking mentations left over from last year's poor diet get washed away with this great muscle food.

The final food group is love. This is a chameleon-like food. It changes to whatever one needs at any one time. It changes on the fly—on a moment's notice. It is strong enough to penetrate every aspect of being and it also radiates out from us toward others. When we really load up on the love foods, our lives truly change in how we look, how we live, how we respond to others, and how we view the world. What is really unique about these foods is that when you share them with others—when you give all these foods away—the karmic weights in life become lighter and lighter and we need less strenuous activity to be successful in changing our lives.

Part Three: Additional Practices

Another interesting thing about these three foods groups is that when you put them on a plate, they run and flow into each other. They have a viscosity to them so that they are sticky. They flow and intermix, combining as one. Whenever anyone picks up the food, it attaches to them, helping to ensure success. They are sweet-tasting, so once you experience a full plate of them, you crave more.

So vow to get back to following your New Year's resolution to change your life. Select the correct foods and get back into the gym of life using the spiritual exercise machines. Over the year you will see a dramatic improvement.

Exercise: Living a Fulfilling Life

The following are ten strong suggestions for living a fulfilling life:

1. Honor the connection you have with everything and everyone in the universe, for we are all one.

2. Treat others as you want to be treated because, ultimately, any action or thought you place on another, you also place on yourself.

3. Offer kind words to everyone you meet, especially those from whom you would normally turn away.

4. Practice mindfulness to stay linked to the here and now instead of the unchangeable past and unknowable future. Every moment is a precious moment.

5. Honor everyone equally.

6. Support the life of all sentient beings. When life is ended for nutritional reasons, give thanks and honor to the animal that offered its life for your benefit.

7. Honor all of your relationships with others.

8. Share what you have with those in need.

9. Be honest. See reality for what it is, without filters or attachments.

10. Reduce consumption of material possessions. Do more with less. Live a simple life. Eat spiritual foods and exercise with spiritual weights.

Part Three: Additional Practices

Thanksgiving Day—The Point of Giving Thanks

Most countries have a holiday set aside for giving thanks. Here in the United States, the Thanksgiving Day holiday is the third Thursday of every November. Unfortunately, the tradition of Thanksgiving has devolved into gorging on food, watching parades and football on TV, and preparing to spend lots of money on Black Friday. Now, a great number of stores are opening from 8 p.m. to midnight on Thanksgiving Day so shoppers don't have to wait to part with their money.

Although it is traditional for families to come together to partake of the feast, how many of them are even thinking about giving thanks for anything? What we really should be giving thanks for on this special day and every day is the opportunity to start anew each day. Be thankful for waking up and experiencing being alive for one more day, and for each day we have the gift of life.

We can choose how that day will be. We may not be able to control the events of the day, but we can control our responses to those events. We can choose to roll with it and call it "all good," or we can fight it and call it "stupid, bad, unfair, unjust, and against me." The exact same events can be given any of these labels depending on how we choose to see it.

So if you want to be genuinely happy, then make a conscious effort to do so. With conscious effort what might be considered a "bad day" can easily be transformed into a "good day."

Be thankful for the opportunity to right any of your past wrongs. Be thankful for others in your life even if the only person you talk to is a sales clerk. Be thankful for all you have and all you have not, today and every day can be happy days of thanks!

Depression

Today, the disease of depression is like a plague. It rages through developed nations virtually unstoppable. It appears to affect people of all race, genders, and creeds. It is worse where there is moderate to extreme wealth and highly evolved systems of communication. Apparently, if we are dirt poor but everyone around us is the same AND we are not exposed to other "opportunities" (i.e., we do not know how the wealthy of the world lives), then we are more content with our lot in life.

However, if we are presented regularly with images of material wealth, others enjoying the "good life," then the knowledge of our "lacking" leads to dissatisfaction and depression. Of course psychologists and psychiatrists will tell you this is a simplistic view and there are many different reasons for depression that are unique to each individual. They say chemical imbalance is the culprit and all we need is the right mix of chemicals and our depression will lift. Just ignore the fact that those miracle cures for depression can often cause diabetes, high blood pressure, liver disease, blindness, even death—but hey! You will be smiling on your way to the grave.

Rather than pop pills, how about doing what comes naturally to humankind? Go back to our "uncivilized" days when we slept under the stars, traveled on foot, and lived off the land. Granted, there are few places in cities today that provide the kind of natural setting required to live naturally.

Our jobs today require us to multi-task with emission-emitting devices connected to our ears, computer monitors sitting less than 36 inches from our eyes, and blasting our hearts and minds with electrical impulses 24/7. Those electrical impulses even blast us through TV computers and smart phones that surround our beds. Even worse, many people insist they cannot sleep without the noise of the TV running all night. The human body just doesn't have a chance; it cannot compete with the forces of technology that drag us down.

An important first step toward good mental health is to unplug. Remove the source of electrical impulses that bombard you. Shut down the "communication system" that tells you what evil and pains the world is constantly inflicting on itself (that is, news broadcasts). Disconnect from the noise. Make time to be still, to be silent, and to quiet your mind. The key to happiness is not in a pill but in a quiet mind. The only way to quiet the mind is to remove stimulation.

Unplug from sound, do not send it directly into your brain through ear buds or headphones. If you absolutely must listen to music through headsets, make sure that only healing instrumentals with soothing tones surround you. Words should only be uplifting and let them take you up with them.

Some people say that silence is unbearable for them because the voices in their head get too loud. There is nothing to drown the voices out. They say listening to the voices only causes a deepening of depression and or paranoia.

None of this is new information. The disease is well-documented and researched around the world. The key to controlling depression is controlling your breath, heartbeat, and thoughts at regular intervals throughout the day. Take a moment to stop, focus on your breath, and slow your heart rate. By spending additional seconds resting at the end of the exhale you can reduce your blood pressure and thereby reduce your heart rate. By focusing on your body's cycle of life, breath, and heartbeat, you can silence the mind. The more you can incorporate this natural state of being into your daily actions, the lighter and happier you will feel. A positive side-effect is that you feel rejuvenated by the calm in your mind instead of fatigued by a drug treatment.

It does not require hours of sitting in long meditations. Just focus on what is at hand in the present moment without allowing your mind to wallow in the past or wander into the future.

The NOW will provide you with what you need to be relaxed and content. It is only in this state that one can be free of depression.

Try it. Really make a strong effort over a period of a week. You will see a marked difference. The longer you practice, the more this natural state of being will once again become natural for you.

All Red Roses

Roses are beautiful. They have a distinct scent, long stems, come in many colors and varieties, and they have thorns—beauty and danger all in one. Very few other flowers have this combination of beauty to attract and thorns to punish.

Unfortunately, there are people who are like roses. They have beautiful appearances, pleasant voices, and usually a compelling story. However, as you get to know them better, you discover their ability to be cutting and mean-spirited. They punish admirers who come too near with thorns that pierce and scratch.

Mean-spiritedness is an interesting description. Typically, if we say that someone is "spirited" that is a complement. It means someone is full of life, energetic, and godly. Qualifiers are frequently used as in "good spirits," "low spirits," or "high spirits," describing a state of mind/body interaction. There are few phrases that have this unique duel meaning. When you preface "spirited" with the adjective "mean," it changes the meaning to describe a person who does things or thinks things that are not in the best interest of others.

Ego-based people are masters of the art of cutting others with their tongues. The effect is more deadly than a fist or a knife. The reason it is more deadly is because the words have the ability to drill into the psyche of the receiver in such a way as to make the receiver believe that they deserve such abuse. With a physical beating, the receiver will become fearful but not necessarily believe they deserved it. Only after many, many repeated physical assaults does the receiver come to believe it is their fault; the other person is justified in abusing them. The most insidious aspect of all types of abusive relationships is the mind/spirit control by the abuser.

How do we know when a relationship has the potential to turn manipulative? Pay attention to your bodily and spiritual reaction when you are near a person. Is there an attraction that you just cannot quite put your finger on? Do you feel as though you are being caught in a vortex and pulled in closer and closer? Is there a whiff of potential danger that makes it exciting, maybe like the thrill of driving a beautiful sports car at speeds well above the legal limit? The danger element is exciting, but you initially do not perceive it as deadly.

When you meet such people—BEWARE! Better yet, turn and RUN! Manipulative and verbally abusive people are much more deadly than someone who is open and up front with their hostilities.

Some fundamental religions exhibit these same characteristics. On the surface, they are welcoming. They make you feel special by their "exclusive" nature. "Only the best can be one of us." Then once they have you, they ask you do to things that are "mean-spirited." No true representatives of a core faith would ever ask another to do something mean-spirited. They could never pollute the body and mind with an unhealthy spirit.

So before you agree to "drink the Kool-Aid" carefully observe the adherents to that religion or philosophy. Do they appear to be roses? Are they offering something that is highly attractive and sweetly scented? Does everyone exhibit strange robotic behavior? Does everyone regurgitate the same thoughts almost mechanically? Are different ideas encouraged or squashed? Does everyone seem a bit too plastic and homogeneous?

If the answer is yes to anyone of those questions, then quickly turn and walk away. The beauty of the false promises will draw you in and the mean-spirited thorns will imprison you by making you doubt your ability to function without them. This is much more than "brain washing." It is "spirit snatching." Move away from the edge of the abyss—now! You have the power to be in control of who you let into your life. Make wise choices early and often. Reassess the people in your life on a regular basis. Ask yourself—is the relationship with him or her still in your best interest and the interest of any children you may have? If not, you do have the power and the right to walk away. If you are being threatened, seek out battered women or men shelters for assistance if the police cannot help you. Only you can take responsibility for moving yourself out of harm's way. Be strong, you can do it.

It's All a Game

Life—it's all a game. Some believe there are winners and losers in life. Those that have the wealth and power—the one percent—they are the "winners." Those that live below the poverty line are the "losers." The vast number of people between the two extremes—well, we might be bluffing to stay in the game. With a couple of good poker hands, we may win the pot and be able to continue playing, or we may fold.

Living in the one percent realm is not without its problems. In many ways, they can become cut off from the rest of the world, typically by choice. Their vision of reality becomes distorted and their ability to relate to normal life becomes challenged. You may scoff at this and say, "I'd like to give life in the one percent a try anyway. I'd rather have the pain of too much money rather than too little."

However, both extremes tend to have the same fears:

- Security. If you are living on the street or in a very poor neighborhood, security is an issue. Robbery, shootings, and home invasions are problems. This is also true for the one percent in their gated communities with security systems and guard dogs.

- Drug usage is a serious problem for both groups. One group's drugs may be a bit purer than the other's, but all of it kills and destroys lives.

- Lack of jobs. The poor typically would like a job but often lack the skills to obtain one. The wealthy don't need them, so both groups have too much time on their hands and lack sources of self-esteem and satisfaction from doing something constructive with their lives.

- Poor health. The poor lack nutritional food and the wealthy become ill because of the richness of their food.

We could go on with these comparisons but what is the point? The point is that moderation is the key to happiness and health—the middle way, as it was so aptly put thousands of years ago by the Buddha.

A recent research study found that an income of $50,000 was the break point at which we are the happiest in the United States. Above that income other issues kick in and we no longer feel as happy.

What if you actively chose to cut your consumption of everything by 50 percent, finding your own middle way, so to speak?

- Drive 50 percent less and walk, ride a bicycle, or take public transportation instead.

- Eat 50 percent less—cutting out those items that are less healthy.

- Spend 50 percent less time plugged into the vast array of available electronics and more time reading and really being present with your family and friends.

- Reduce busy work by 50 percent and more time spent in meditation or meditative activities like gardening.

- Buy and consume 50 percent less material goods and save the money for a rainy day, retirement, or helping others.

Part Three: Additional Practices

The game of life would be so much easier to play and be so much more rewarding if we would only cut everything we do and consume by half.

A great place to start is by reducing the amount of complaining you do by 50 percent and increase your listening by the same amount.

just smile and laugh at the situations that would typically trigger a complaint. Gradually extend this to two days a week, then three until the complaining behavior is extinguished. You will discover the joy of being relieved of this burden.

Go through all you own and clear out everything you have not used in the last year or two. Donate it to a charity so that the items can benefit others and DO NOT replace those items with more things.

Talk to your neighbors beyond just waving hello. Get to know them for who they are. Help each other out.

Find a sangha or spiritual community; this is a group of people with whom you can discuss ways of spiritual growth and development. Find a mentor, a teacher with whom you can relate. Find your connection to that which connects us all.

This is the way of the middle path. This is the way to contentment. Contentment breeds happiness. Change the rules of your game and you change your life.

Ring of Fire

On the evening of May 20, 2012, a rare annular eclipse occurred. This is a ring of light that is created as the new moon, passing between Earth and sun in exact alignment that blocks most, but not all, of the sun's disc. An annular eclipse is different from a total solar eclipse, in that the moon in an annular eclipse appears too small to cover the sun completely. This leaves what appears to be a ring of fire around the moon. The eclipse was seen in a narrow path crossing the west from Texas to Oregon then arcing across the northern Pacific Ocean to Tokyo, Japan.

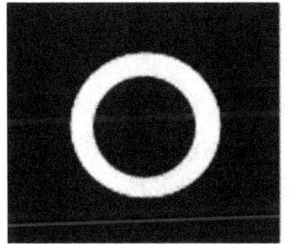
Author's Rendition

What might be the significance of this event? How might we interpret it other than just the passing of one astral body in front of another? Let us say that the sun represents an individual spirit—you. The dark moon represents all of the learning experiences of everyday life. We all have an inherent glow, which is our Buddha-nature, essence, soul, or spirit. It is stunningly beautiful, full, and complete, without imperfections. However, the events in our lives sometimes pass by us in such a manner as to obscure our vision of our inherent shining selves. The full glow of our Buddha-nature still encompasses the obstacles and shines around them, thereby providing an even more spectacular view of ourselves when we are actively working with the teachings. As we live the teachings, the obstacles gradually pass away and the whole of our Buddha-nature shines once again.

Mudra—Have No Fear

Mudra is a term that is used to refer to the position of hand placements in Buddhist images. Each position has a different meaning. A commonly seen image of Shakyamuni Buddha shows the Buddha with his hands in the standard "No Fear" posture. Let's examine what the mudra means. The upward right hand is interpreted as "Have no fear." The lower left hand facing outward and down means "Your needs will be met."

When the image is placed facing you, the fingers of Buddha's right hand are extended upward to draw on the assistance of the universe. Energy flows from the universe down through the fingers and out the palms of the hand directly into your heart. The lower left hand also shows the palms flat facing forward. The fingers are pointing downward, grounding you to the earth. The energy of the Buddha (universal energy) is aimed downward to stabilize you and out the palms of the hand into your heart. By merely being in front of the image, you passively absorb the energy and it will help to remove your fears of relinquishing attachment, and provide you with energy to meet your needs.

You can also actively use this mudra for yourself.

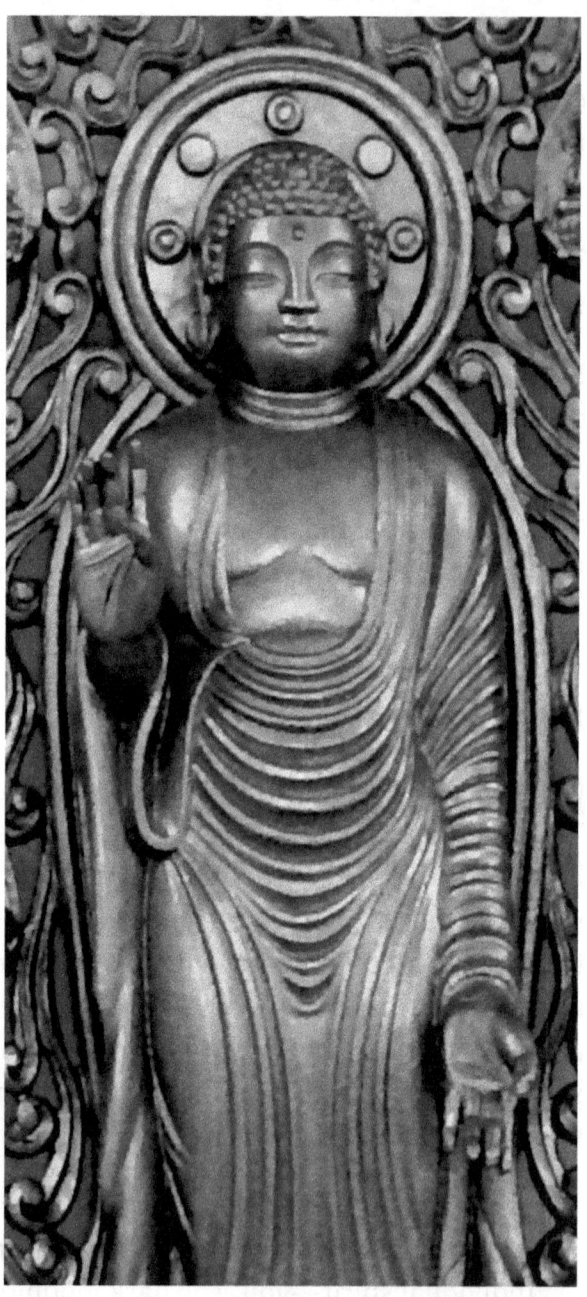

Photo by Jane Perri

Exercise: Have No Fear

First, sit relaxed, in a meditational posture in front of the image. Raise your hands the same way as the Buddha, right hand up, left hand facing down with both palms forward.

- Visualize the energy coming from the right hand of Buddha to your right hand. Run it through your arm into your heart and then into your left arm and out your left hand, back to the Buddha's left hand.

- Notice that you are creating a figure eight, the sign for infinity, as the energy exchanges between the hands. This energy has always been and always will be available for your use.

- What you are doing is bringing in universal energy to help you to extinguish your fears: fears of moving forward on your path, fear of not having what you need in your material or spiritual lives. The energy runs through and activates your heart, turning it into compassionate energy. Energy in and of itself has no value, hue, or flavor. By running it through your heart, it transforms into compassionate energy.

- When you visualize sending the compassionate energy out of yourself and into the left hand of the Buddha, you will stabilize yourself in the earth energy.

Doing this visualization is only one-half of the process. This is just to get you charged up, so to speak.

When you go out into the world, out of your contemplative state, you can use this mudra to calm your fears and provide for your own needs. Here is the second half of the process:

- After you are charged up with universal transmitted energy, put your hands into the Have No Fear mudra, with the right hand upright about the level of your shoulder and the left arm downward. Palms should be facing forward on both hands.

- Tap into the universal energy with your right hand and run the energy into your heart to condition it for compassion.

- Next, send out compassionate energy into the world though your palms while grounding yourself to the earth energy with fingers pointed towards the earth.

Note: The energy going out is to help OTHERS fulfill their needs. It is ONLY when you help others that you will help yourself. It is like running electricity through a light bulb. You have electricity coming in at one point (right hand) crossing a wire (heart) and going to another port or receptacle (others). The bulb does not work if the wire disconnects from the receiving port. If you try to keep all the energy for yourself and not extend it to others, it is just like breaking the circuit in the light bulb. Your life will not glow. Yes, you will still have the physical shell—just like the glass of the bulb, but it will not radiate. It will not be of any use or substance. The glass of your body will easily shatter. When you share the connection with others, helping others, the energy will warm your own body and spirit, and you will glow with compassion.

This is your purpose in life. It is the purpose of all of us. We are here together to help each other, to support one another, and to ground each other. Try it—it works.

Living Life Easy

There are dozens of web sites that you can find that would like to sell you their special program on how to live an easy life. Most are "get-rich-quick" schemes designed to make the purveyor of the site richer than you.

There are ways to live the easy life that do not cost you a cent. The difference, however, is in the definition of easy. "Living life easy" is not the same as "living the easy life."

"Living the easy life" implies that you have sufficient financial resources, that you do not need to work, or that you work minimally. This may be "easy" but it is not a recipe for happiness. In fact, it will most likely bring you unhappiness because your self-esteem is often bolstered by your accomplishments and hard work that you can be proud of doing. If everything were available to us without effort, we would no longer value the small (or large) things in life that once brought us pleasure.

"Living life easy" is different. It does not involve money, it relates to how you personally struggle with your everyday existence. Some people are depressed, others anxious, stressed out, or just plain unhappy. These are not easy conditions to deal with on a long-term basis. Even if you indulge in the plethora of legal and illegal drugs, or alcohol to numb you, the "dis-ease" still may haunt you.

So what is the magic bullet? What can replace the dis-ease with positive or at least neutral feelings? The answer is non-attachment—letting go.

Let go of the past events in your life—they no longer serve you. They only prevent you from living fully in the present. Let go of your fears for the future. The future hasn't happened yet and the more you fear it, the more likely you will cause what you fear to happen by giving it energy and attention. If you stop obsessing over it, it will vanish.

Let go of anger. Remove swear words from your vocabulary. They have strong negative energy that is sticky and gooey, which makes it hard to release the anger. Replace them with blessings instead.

Let go of the need for revenge. Forgiveness is one of the best medicines there is for past pain. Try it; there are only good results without any negative side-effects.

Let go of your need to control every detail in your life and the lives of those around you. It cannot be done anyway, so why waste the energy and boost stress levels needlessly—yours and others around you.

Let go of expectations. Let things unfold in life without you trying to script it in advance. If you do not expect anything, then when you get nothing, there are no emotional responses to disturb your calm state of being.

Let go of taking on other people's stressors as your own—it is not always about you. In fact, other people's stressors are rarely about you so don't make them yours. Don't you have enough of your own?

Let go of needing to be right all of the time, it is impossible anyway. Let go of needing to be superior to others; we are all equal, you are just stressing yourself out trying.

Do take time regularly to be silent and calm. Meditate daily, if only for a few minutes at a time. Your mind will benefit from stopping the chatter for awhile.

Be grateful for all you have and all you have not. Learn to say "thank you ten, twenty, thirty times a day, and at the end of the day, let gratitude for that day be the last thought in your mind.

Non-attachment to life's events does not mean that you don't care for those in your life. It simply means that you are comfortable with change and realize that all things will change, so there is no sense in investing in them. Life will play out as it is intended to whether you stress out, get depressed over it, or just let it go.

By simply replacing attachment with gratitude, you will find your life will be immensely easier and more joyful. All others in your life will appreciate the change and it will help them to be calmer, too. A wonderful supportive cycle will be set in motion as you positively influence others and they in kind, reinforce your changes. It is a lot cheaper and healthier than taking medications, and the side effects are wonderful.

Exercise: Replacing Attachment with Gratitude

Contemplate the following questions:

Do you focus on living in the moment? If so, how do you do it?

What is your habit with the usage of swear words? Do you notice a difference in your emotional level when you use them?

What aspects of your life and relationships do you habitually try to control? How can you let go of the need to control?

What expectation did you have in a relationship that caused you problems?

Part Three: Additional Practices

Do you consciously (or unconsciously) hold others to your expectations? Can you explain why you do this?

Do you have thoughts about being superior or inferior to others? If so, what do you consciously do when you get them? If you do not compare yourself with others, why do you think you have been able to avoid this trap?

Do you consider yourself to be a grateful person? What is your evidence? If not, why not?

When is it difficult for you to say thank you and to be a grateful person? Why is this?

Do you feel an energetically charged when you are grateful? Do you like this feeling?

Homework

- Go for one full week without trying to control situations and others around you. Keep a journal of your progress. If you find that you get sucked in, then write how you might be able to do something different when the situation presents itself again.

- If you can't do it for a week, then try it for a day.

Working this exercise, one day at a time, until you master your attachment is the key to success. As stated earlier, replacing attachment with gratitude, will lead you to an easier and more joyful life.

Journal Record of Practicing to Control Situations (Add more pages as needed.)

It's Not Summertime Everywhere

Ah, summertime. The sun finally begins to warm the earth. The flowers are in full bloom along with seasonal allergies. Kids are out of school, on the playgrounds, and in swimming pools. This is the reality for only a portion of our earth's inhabitants. Those in the southern hemisphere are in the dead of winter, while those in the north are frolicking on the beaches. Of course, for those that live in the equatorial bands, climate does not have the broad temperature swings at all. It's always summertime hot there.

This is representative of so many things in life; my reality is not your reality. What I see is not what you see. What I feel is not what you feel. My reaction to events is not your reaction to the exact same event. You know what? This is all okay.

Because of our biological make up, it is impossible for two people to be exactly alike in every way—even monozygotic twins do not think the same—even if they do dress alike. So why then, do parents get so upset when their children adopt a different spiritual practice or political belief from their own? Oftentimes, the parents take it as a sign of personal failure. "Where did I go wrong, that Jamie is so darn different?!!!"

Fear, anger, and hatred for those who hold different ideas from us has become a pandemic disease, not just in the United States, but also in most countries around the world today. We in the United States are not acting out as violently as elsewhere, but people are dying here just because they believe differently from some unstable people with guns or bombs. Ego has wrought the destruction of our fellow inhabitants, even before we learned to walk upright. The great apes show the same hostile behaviors toward their own kind as humans do. This behavior is indeed animalistic.

To achieve the "peace on earth" that everyone says they want, we ALL, on both sides of the divide, must change our views and attitudes. The change we must have is not to take the opposite view, but simply to allow other views to exist and be okay with it. "You are you, I am me, and that is okay." This is certainly not a new or groundbreaking idea. Pacifists and reasonable people throughout the millennia have used it to discourage war—without success.

Today, more than at any time in our human past, the planet is filled with hatred in a way that never existed before. It is of epidemic proportions and innocent men, women, and children are dying for no reason other than ego. We are not in a great world war but the one-on-one violence is like a cancer, growing in every direction. Some individual or group believes he, she, or they must have their way; they must have the power to impose their will on others.

So what can we do to make a difference in reducing the pain and violence levels of the world? Most people throw up their hands and declare they can do nothing, but this is not true. Because we are all connected energetically, the energy we send out does ripple, in kind, to others. If we are hateful, hatred radiates out from us, colors everything gray, and dampens the positive energy of the world.

When you are still and your mind at rest without chatter, without judgment, anger, or fear, you naturally become a beacon of light and radiate neutralizing energy. It is critical for the survival of our human race that we neutralize the dominating forces of hate, anger, and fear.

The more often you do not react to confrontations in your everyday life, the more you neutralize them. A reaction needs an opposite reaction to continue the momentum. When no reaction occurs, the sender may escalate the negativity, in an attempt to trigger the response to feed on, but continued baiting will not be effective if we do not engage. Remain detached, neutral—do not get sucked into the dark hole.

This is difficult to do, but it is a practice. Every time we succeed in not responding, the negativity of the universe reverses just a bit. The impact it has on you and the other person is much greater. To be the person you want to be—to bring "peace on earth" or just to your family or self—do not engage. Non-engagement means do not get into the verbal (or physical) sparring, but let the statements go by and fizzle out on their own. It is only when you give it energy by responding to it that it will grow in strength and negativity. So combat negativity with non-engagement.

The next step is to send loving compassionate acceptance to that person energetically, even if you cannot do it verbally. Just like the Grinch who stole Christmas, the hearts of all people who have been damaged by their ego, can be healed. "Peace on earth" is possible and it starts with you and me.

Exercise: Palpable Emotional Output

- Ask someone to help you with this experiment. Sit opposite your partner.

- Ask that person to recall a scenario that they have been in—one that caused him or her extreme anger to the point where they wanted to take revenge. Ask them to try to remember as many details as possible. They do not need to verbalize this, just think about the event.

- As they are doing this, see if you can feel energy radiate from him or her. If the exercise is done in a dim light, you might even be able to see a reddish glow from them. This is the emotional energy changing their aura.

- Now ask your partner to think of a situation in which he or she showed extreme compassion, where they went out of their way, to help another person in need. Ask that they recall as many details as possible, including how they felt during and after the event.

- Again try to sense an energy radiating from him or her. You might be able to see a greenish glow from your partner in a dim light.

- Did you a sense the difference in the energetic output from the two events?

- Reverse roles and repeat the exercise.

Show and Shine Drive-In

Summertime typically brings out the Show and Shine Drive-Ins with old car enthusiasts showing off their winter restoration work. The drive-in usually brings in throngs of people who reminisce about days gone by, as well as younger people who long to own one of the hot rods to show their manhood. These drive-ins and also antique shops serve an important function in our material world. They remind us that newer is not always better.

Today's marketers entice us to buy, buy, buy. We have become a disposable society. Products are built to last only a short while and then be replaced to keep the engines of the economy running. We are told that spending beyond our means with credit is desirable, and even our patriotic duty.

All of the buying and disposing creates a huge footprint that harms the earth. Our landfills are overflowing with lightly used items that could have been repurposed. Recycling is critical for the earth's survival. However, the type of recycling I am talking about is that which has you reusing items for longer periods of time, before throwing them out.

Attachments, cravings to always having the newest of this, the best of that, the same as his or hers is damaging to the human psyche and to the physical body. It creates an artificial sense of need that becomes indistinguishable from desire. "I need a new pair of shoes." The fact that I already have two dozen pairs in my closet is irrelevant. Children are taught from a very young age that more is better. They are indulged with dozens and dozens of toys, so much so that their rooms are overflowing with them. The kids don't play with them because there are simply too many, but parents and family misread it as they must not like them, so they buy more and more and more.

All of these material things then produce a need to protect them from theft, so a whole new layer of stress is artificially created.

Simplify your life! Break the bondage that desire and attachment have on you. When you are happy with what you have, you spend less, leaving more money available to pay off accumulated debt or save for the future. This also relieves stress.

It is difficult to focus on developing your spiritual life when you have to work increased hours or two jobs to pay for your material excesses.

You can't take your materials possessions with you into the next life, but you do take your spiritual development. The level of development, at which you end one life, is where you begin your next adult life. So the phrase "you can't take it with you" is correct in regards to material possessions but not spiritual growth; therefore, all of our efforts to accumulate are misplaced. If the ownership of jewels and fancy cars do not contribute to the development of our spiritual growth, then they are unimportant.

Many of the Christian TV evangelists say that monetary wealth is a sign that God loves you. This could not be further from the truth. Money has nothing to do with love of anything but money and it is an illusion. If you want more, be satisfied with less. This is absolutely critical in our development on our path to enlightenment and spiritual growth.

Again, if you want more, be satisfied with less. Once you have internalized this concept, once you begin to live by this, you will be amazed how your life will change. Your stress levels will reduce and your happiness quotient will rise. It will be as if you have just learned another language and stepped into a new culture, because you have. A culture that is satisfied, delighted, and content with what is, instead of craving what is not. There will be a new freedom from stress and doubt that lightens the load on your shoulders and heart. You will feel lighter and freer and it all begins with living a simpler life.

Begin today by not buying something. Put that money in a jar or box. Save it for your spiritual future.

Moving into a New Home

The physical act of moving into a new home or apartment is always stressful and difficult. Here are the steps:

1. First there is the decision to leave what is familiar and comfortable. Even if you don't particularly like where you are currently residing, at least you know what to expect.

2. Then there is the job of packing. This is physically difficult but mentally even more so because within the period of a few days or weeks you revisit every aspect of your life in that residence. You need to decide what mementos to keep and which to throw away. Oftentimes, memories of specific events are triggered by a memento that can be either pleasant or otherwise.

3. Next is the physical strain of loading the moving vehicle(s), stacking your life in boxes and padded wraps, carefully squashed down into small compact spaces, and driving away.

4. You still have to return to clean out the last residue of your life in the old place and throw it away.

5. Arriving at your new location offers hopes and dreams of a better life, a happier life, a fresh start. As we unpack our things and place them in their new location of honor, we think about how our lives are being rearranged too.

This scenario plays out frequently throughout life. It marks major transitions, defines periods, and helps us to grow. It puts brackets around periods like new chapters in a book, fresh start, but still some continuance of the thread of your prior existence.

What do you want to carry forward? What do you prize about yourself? What do you want to change? The move offers opportunities for fresh breaks. It can bring closure to old habits that no longer serve your higher interest or your spiritual self.

Take this opportunity to clean out those habits that are self-defeating and destructive. Take this opportunity to renew your vows to love yourself and those with whom you live. Take this opportunity to view your life from an angle different from where you have been. You have already stepped outside of your comfort zone, so make good use of your courage and honestly assess where you have been and where you want to go with your life.

Change is good. Change is refreshing. Change is inevitable. Don't waste the opportunity to really clean house—of your heart and mind of old habits.

Rejoice in the service of your new life. It is filled with possibility that you have not yet imagined.

Coffee, Tea, or Me, or Ten Steps to a Better You

A great number of people, if not most adults in western culture, have developed the practice of drinking a cup of tea or coffee each morning to get them moving. Some use soft drinks or energy drinks for the same purpose—caffeine! That morning jolt tells you that you are alive. There is even something called the caffeine headache for the truly addicted that can be cured only with a good dosage of the life-supporting substance.

Starbucks may not like this idea but what if everyone replaced this practice with a morning contemplative period instead? Instead of getting up early to brew your "cup of Joe," or to stop by Starbucks or other caffeine drive-thru, why not position yourself instead in a comfortable chair for 5 minutes and reflect on the upcoming day. This is not to suggest that you go over your grocery or "to-do" list for the day. There is no use in starting off stressing yourself out. Instead, reflect on how you will respond to the world today.

Exercise: Ten Steps to a Better You

When you consciously set your emotional course for the day, it will always run more smoothly. Follow these steps to a more awakened day:

1. Create a sacred space for regular usage. It is best if the space is in an area that you walk past on your way to start the day. A nook in your bedroom works much better than a corner in the living room.

   Place in the space a straight-back chair or stool, something not too comfortable, something to support a straight back. Also place a small table in the space; it need not be more than a foot wide, even less will do. On the table place a small candle and an image of a great sage that you admire for their philosophy and ethical conduct. It could be a religious leader but it does not have to be. You could use a symbol for peace or love, too. The candle is to bring in energy, light, and focus to your mind. Electrical lights should not be used for this as they are inert. Select an image or object that will provide you with direction and aspirational growth.

2. With the candle in front of the image, sit upright in a relaxed but straight-backed posture. Focus your eyes one-half to three-quarters closed on the candle and image. Your position should be such that all the energy will radiate into your heart. Visualize breathing the energy in through your heart.

3. Then say aloud:

   > I release all my anger.
   > I release all my fear.
   > I release all my prejudice.
   > I release all my separation.
   > I am acceptance.
   > I am compassion.
   > I am love.
   > In all my thoughts and actions, I am one with all. I trust that all this is true.

4. Then just allow the calm sweet energy to flood into and through you. Fully charge yourself up. After a few moments, ask for the spiritual growth you would like that day. Examples:

- "Today I will practice patience and acceptance. I will be calm and respond calmly to the days' events. Kindness will replace anger."

- "I will respond today with compassionate wisdom to all situations instead of material gain, power, or ego."

- "I will see love in everyone I meet today, instead of prejudice or distain."

- "I will relate to everyone as my equal, which they are, instead of feeling superior or less than."

5. The point here is to phrase everything in a positive affirmative format, not negative as in "I will not..." Our mind naturally will reject being told not to do something even if we give the command to ourselves.

6. Focus on a single thought or action for the day. More than that will be too difficult and nonproductive. Experience the statement. How does it sound? How does it feel? How does it taste? How does it move through you? How does it resonate out of you? Absorb it into your cellular being and vow to follow the course of action for that day.

7. End the session in asking for guidance and giving thanks for the opportunity to grow that day.

8. Hold the action plan for the day in your heart and mind all day and revisit it often. You might even want to write it down on a slip of paper and put it into your pocket. Then when you feel it there throughout the day, it will remind you to refocus and re-center yourself.

9. In the evening, as the last thing you do before you crawl into bed, reseat yourself in your sacred space, relight your candle, and give thanks for the day. Give thanks for the lessons learned and thanks for those who learned from you today.

10. Finish off with simply allowing the love energy to flow from the heart of your image into yours.

This centering period need not be long, 5 minutes both morning and night on a regular basis will change your life for the better—guaranteed. You cannot get this benefit from coffee!

Bicycling in the Snow

Avid bicyclists are a hardy bunch. They are typically passionate about riding. Their conversations will almost always include a reference to the activity or life style. They believe that they are doing something good for the planet by burning muscle fuel instead of fossil fuel and they are correct. Many will ride in all four seasons as long as they possibly can and this includes riding in the snow. Vacations are frequently planned around two-wheel road trips.

Bicycling, in addition to being a great hobby, sport, and form of transportation, is an easy analogy for life.

A child does not automatically know how to ride a bicycle. Even with tricycles, they start out walking it or scooting themselves along before they get the hang of putting their feet on the pedals and pumping.

In the same way, when we first begin to "ride" the teachings of a spiritual practice, we have to have trust that the teachings will carry us. We keep one foot planted in disbelief as we gradually, carefully, put the other on the step that rises up from entry- to mid- to advanced-level teachings.

Once we master the motion of pedaling, we can tear around on our hot wheels or tricycle at great speed, staying low to the ground and moving fast.

As we begin our foray into the teachings, there is typically an early stage that we are ecstatic about finding something that on the surface appears that it might suit us well. So, we hungrily devour book after book on the topic, reading an assortment of authors and sages, with no particular direction. Regardless of the religion, there are thousands of titles written that offer a wealth of knowledge and opinion, oftentimes giving conflicting information.

As we mature in our abilities on the tricycle, our parents decide it is time to move up a level to a bicycle. Since finding our balance can be difficult, they put training wheels on it for us. Much the same as when we decide which form of a particular religion attracts us, we seek out a teacher that gives us a specific sacred text to focus on. There are primary sacred texts for every religion and then some "training wheel" books that interpret it for us.

Once we have mastered our balance and found our center, our parents remove the training wheels. In just the same way, our mentor removes the supporting texts and encourages us to delve deeply in the primary sacred text with all of its hidden meanings.

As we grow, we move to larger bicycles, gradually moving farther away from the center of our balance of gravity so we get a different view of the world from a higher perspective point or advantage point. The same is true in our quest for deeper spiritual understanding. We must continue to practice at increasingly higher levels, to understand fully the world around us. The higher up we go, the clearer the line of sight.

As we age from child, to adolescent, to teen, oftentimes we will double up on a bike, putting a friend on the seat or handle bars as we pedal. It is great fun but harder to pedal. We gladly do it as the ride is often filled with laughter, creating lasting memories of the bonding experience.

In much the same way, when we bring a friend along or develop new friendships in our spiritual quest, it becomes more fun and provides a sense of family and belonging. We share our experiences and make new memories together as we continue to learn and practice together. Sometimes when we are down, our spiritual friends and teachers carry us. When they are down, we carry them.

The more we ride a bike, the more it becomes a way of life. It is no longer just a form of transportation; it becomes our way of breathing air, of strengthening our muscles, and improving our overall health.

When we look at the great spiritual traditions of the world, we see that the most central teachings of each tradition are essentially the same: love yourself and others, have compassion for all, recognize and understand who you really are, the central spiritual essence and our connection/sameness with the divine life force. When we study the teachings in earnest, the study gives way to practice, and practice becomes a way of living, effortless and seamless in our lives. We then move from being the student to being the mentor—just like the young adult becomes the parent who teaches their child to ride.

Once we have incorporated the teachings completely into our lives, they are available to us whenever we need them to overcome the steep hill we are riding up or when we are pedaling in snow that bogs us down.

By using our toolkit to adjust the chains and add more gears to make it easier to climb, we grow in our maturity. Using the positive, loving tools of our faith, we can repair any flat tire that temporarily waylays us. We can fine-tune our thinking that helps move us up mountains more easily. So don't just sit by the side of the road if something breaks on your bike—get out your toolkit, use it, and move on.

The rest that you take while you are figuring out the repair can be just what you need to continue your journey, and thereby return refreshed and renewed. By using your spiritual toolkit, you gain greater insight into your true nature, to what is really important—living and breathing, who we really are, as we really are, our Buddha-nature, our god center, our oneness with the divine, our universal life force energy. Whatever name you are comfortable in calling it—it is all one and the same. You are it, I am it, he, she, they are it, we are all it, together as one. When our spiritual practice has been mastered, it becomes our life practice and that is when bicycling in the snow is as easy as riding in the sunlight. Become one with the teachings.

Part Three: Additional Practices

Exercise: Developing Your Spiritual Practice

Write your personal story of the growth process in your spiritual development.

Part Three: Additional Practices

What was your life like before the spark?

What incentivized you to seek something else?

What have been your "mountains" and "snow" along the way?

What are you doing to keep yourself moving ahead?

Who are the people on your "handle bars" that are sharing the "ride" with you? Why did you select them? What will you gain from their companionship?

What words of wisdom do you have for those that are just getting their "training wheels"?

Part Three: Additional Practices

Is Truth Situational?

George Washington was famous for saying, "I cannot tell a lie, I cut down the cherry tree." Honesty is a characteristic that everyone says they value above all else, even criminals that lie for a living insist on honesty among thieves. However, it is extremely rare to find someone who is honest all the time. There is a qualifying type called "a little white lie," that most people believe to be acceptable.

Is it okay to lie to spare someone's feelings? For example, is it okay to be honest if someone asks you to give an opinion on something that if you were honest, it would hurt his or her feelings? Is it okay to tell the little white lie to protect that person? The spiritually correct answer is—maybe. Deflection is a better response than outright lying. Instead of saying "the outfit makes you look fat," you can say "the color really brings out your eyes." Brutal honesty that will cause unhappiness when the outcome is not of dire importance is more harmful than honest deflection that is uplifting rather than defeating. In all other situations honesty is, as they say, "the best policy."

Occasionally, we will meet a person who never says an unkind word about anyone. These people are highly sought after by others to be friends. It is not that they are well-practiced in the art of deception, but that they understand the art of compassion. This skill involves the ability to find good in all situations and in all people. Even a murderer can be loving to his or her child. Each time we recognize the good in someone, it encourages that person to try to live up to that positive image. It appears to be our nature to "live up to" whatever the important people in our lives repeatedly say to us. If our parents tell us, "You are stupid and will never amount to anything," this thought will worm its way into our subconscious and forever cause us to doubt ourselves unless we actively work to prevent it. Parents can cause permanent damage to their children with careless words. We never know how others will interpret our comments. We all have memories of careless comments we made and wished we could take back or were said to us and have never been forgotten. How much better the world would be if instead of remembering negative views of ourselves, we all remember positive and uplifting views of ourselves.

When we feel honored and accepted, we are not violent. When we feel worthy, we value others. When we are uplifted by others, then we naturally respond by passing the loving support on to others. When many people in a group, neighborhood, or community uplift and support each other, the vibrational rate of the world rises a bit and every inhabitant of the earth lives a bit more comfortably. So, do your part and be supportive of those you encounter each day. Make the first thought that pops into your mind upon meeting someone, be positive not negative. Be affirming and supportive when you can and be neutral at other times. Become that person whom others admire for never saying a bad word about anyone. Do your part to raise the vibrational rate of the world. You will be happier and those around you will be happier, which in turn will reinforce your happiness. Let's all live together a little easier

Sticking to Something that Matters

Do you have a principle or belief that makes up the core of who you are? Do you have a guiding philosophy that is your light to show you the way through the murkiness of life? Such core beliefs are important for our personal navigational compasses.

The core belief does not have to be religious in nature, but optimistically it is moral and ethical at the very least. Hopefully, the philosophy is not the "M" word: MONEY. Hopefully, it is something that matters and sustains you.

Everyone should write his or her own personal mission, vision, and value statements. When you clearly define your purpose, it provides sign posts for you on the path in life.

The first step, however, is to figure out what you value. If your values are of a higher nature, above the common material pursuit, you will more likely be content in life. If your values are to be wealthy, popular, powerful, or to have status or fame, then you are setting yourself up for disappointment. These earthly addictions are just that—addictions. If that is your focus, no matter how much you obtain of any one of them, it will never be enough.

If your core values are on acting with honesty, integrity, being content with who you are and what you have, then happiness will follow.

Mission statements answer the age-old existential question, "Why am I here?" This question has plagued man since the beginning of time, but it does not have to plague you—figure it out! To do that takes the investment of time and focus. It's not something that you pull out of a thought box and claim as your own.

Where to start?

Exercise: Develop Your Personal Mission, Vision, and Value Statements

Set aside a block of time at least 3 or 4 hours to start, and the rest of the week to ponder and tweak it.

1. Find a quiet space where you will not be interrupted. Place a candle on the table to help you focus. If there is an image or symbol of a particular person that exemplifies one who "walks their talk," put that on the table, too.

2. Begin with a meditation and grounding that opens the channels from the universe and earth. Do some deep cleansing breaths and begin.

Part Three: Additional Practices

3. What are your guiding principles? These are principles that you hold dear, actively try to live up to, and do not violate.

4. Write these down! It is best to write the initial draft by hand to feel the process.

    a. Examine your life. What has given you a sense of connection with others in the past?

    b. We are on this earth to help ourselves through helping others. What is it that you can do for others? Start with very specific things you can do and then write a summary statement that encompasses the spirit of the services.

Part Three: Additional Practices

    c. How will you carry out this service—incorporate your values and your guiding principles?

    d. Who is it that you want to serve? Most people would include immediate family members, but extend out beyond this small circle. Every person on this earth is part of your extended family. Which of them can you help?

    e. What personal tools have you developed over the years? What are your skills, your gifts? How can you best use those gifts to serve?

5. After you have written out the answers, then meditate again and sit with your responses and reflections. Know that whatever you write today is an organic living document and that the specific details will change. As you grow in your service, you

Part Three: Additional Practices

will learn so much more that you will want to incorporate into your responses and reflections.

6. Write a paragraph of 5 to 6 lines that pulls all your answers together, and then simplify it down to two sentences. This is the first draft of your mission statement. Feel free to scratch out and revise your work.

7. The vision statement is your target goal in life. At the end of your life, what do you want to reflect back on and say, "I did __ well." Again, this should be based on higher goals, not material and earthly attachments. It should stem from your mission in life; it is you completely fulfilling your mission. What will you do? This statement can be a page long and have many details. If you are going to win an award for your great accomplishment, what would the newspaper article say about you?

8. Meditate again on all you have written.

Part Three: Additional Practices

9. Quickly write down thoughts that came to you in the meditation.

10. Tweak all three statements from insight gained from the meditation.

11. Type everything up on a computer or hand write them. Polish the grammar and edit it again as the thoughts come to you.

12. Post all three documents in a place where you will see them regularly—your kitchen cabinet, refrigerator door, or bathroom mirror. Over the course of the next week—live with them, contemplate them, examine your heart. Do they feel right? If not, make adjustments again.

13. Once you have these maps to guide you, making choices in life becomes easy. Simply ask yourself, "Will this choice lead me toward or away from my goals?" As you move through various stages in your life, revisit your goals periodically to see if they have changed. Update the goals, values, mission, and vision statements as needed.

By sticking to this ritual, your life will improve. Your level of contentment will soar. The lives of those you serve as well as your own will be blessed.

What is the Purpose of Life?

What is the purpose of life? Man has been asking this question since he began walking upright. The answer has had various responses depending on the philosophical slant of the respondent.

The true answer is that the purpose of life is the same for each of us when we first come back into a body from the other side. With each new transmigration, we vow we will do better to live up to that purpose and to set an example for others. Unfortunately, the vast majority fail at least in part.

The foundational purpose of life is to learn to be one with our true spiritual self. Our human instincts push us to behave in ways that is not in keeping with our essence. What is our essence? Love is our essence, pure energetic love of the most compassionate kind.

When we learn to see the world through the eyes of our compassionate essence, we behave much differently. We treat others and ourselves much differently than when we see the world through human eyes.

Human eyes see others as threats. If others get more, then we must get less. We see the world as a win-lose game. This sets the stage for fear, greed, oppression, jealousy, and all of the other human traits that do nothing but cause harm and sadness. We think only of ourselves or maybe we extend our protection to our immediate family and close friends, but no further.

When we see the world through essence eyes, we see no need for competition; we see no need for material gain. Greed and jealousy are not factors; they do not even enter our thoughts because we are content in ourselves and have no need for false physical symbols of "success" or "self-actualization." It is through your "unthoughtful" acts of compassion that your self-actualization is expressed. I say "unthoughtful" because the actions occur without premeditated thought. They are spontaneous and filled with compassion. We do things because it is the natural thing to do, the loving thing to do, not because our actions will result in placing us higher on the material food chain or give us more power and status.

When we understand the true meaning of life—to manifest who we really are and not our almost clownish human images—then we are living out the true meaning of life. We must become one in mind, body, and essence. Our thoughts and actions must occur without the purpose of gaining anything. We think and do the compassionate thing just because that is natural to us.

Very few people are able to manifest their true essence at all times. We allow glimmers of our essence to show through at various times in our lives but not on a sustained level. This is our challenge. This is the challenge we set for ourselves each time we transmigrate into a new body.

Now is the time to go within and try to find the purity, strength, and compassion of your essence and break free from the human jail that confines it. You/we are much greater than we project. As long as we allow our humanness to dictate our thoughts and actions, we will suffer. When we allow our essence to navigate us through life, we live a life of contentment that cannot help but bring us joy. Joy for ourselves and all those we encounter.

Now is the time to stop the chatter in your mind and listen to the messages of the common, single, united, communal essence that we all share. We are all parts of the same essence. Once we tune our human minds into that essence, we no longer will have need for oral communication; we will naturally be able to communicate essence-to-essence. We will truly be "on the same wavelength" without having to go into deep meditation to do it. This type of communication—thought passage—requires more than just one enlightened person. To do this, we need to cultivate the compassionate nature of not only ourselves, but others too.

It is easiest to start with children under the age of six or seven, before their essence becomes fully ensconced into the human body. Maybe this is why we are naturally kind, gentle, and compassionate with children. There is a flicker of memory that is ignited in the presence of a child. We need to learn to extend that reflexive compassionate attitude and behavior to everyone at all times. "Just do it" and the behavior will become habitual. Your behavior will change your thought patterns, which will in turn reinforce your behavior. Now is the time for change. Now is the time to live your true purpose. Now is the time to find your meaning in life. Are you ready? Trigger the domino effect in yourself and your circle of influence. No time is better than now.

Be the Wave of Compassion

In the previous section, we talked about compassion being part of the purpose of life. We talked about the fact that we all are part of the same universal life source. So, are we in anyway unique and distinctive?

The answer is yes and no. We can use the analogy of waves in the oceans to explain. All bodies of salt water are connected. The mighty Pacific meets with the Atlantic and becomes indistinguishable as to where one ends and the other begins. This is like the universal life force energy, the consciousness or repository for all consciousness generated since the beginning of time.

Everywhere along the surface of the great body of water, we find waves. The waves are of varying height, width, length, duration, and form. Each one has its own shape and behavior pattern that at first glance may appear to all be the same. They rise from the forces of the wind, grow to peak height, then fall down and rejoin the ocean body. However, each wave is different; while it rises above the ocean level, it returns to its oneness with the ocean body a short time later—only to rise again in a new life.

This illustrates the cycle of life, death, transmigration, and rebirth that we all repeatedly go through until we step off the karmic wheel and no longer have a need for rebirth.

We awaken to our true nature—our oneness with all there is. With this understanding or as a result of this understanding, our thoughts and behavior patterns change too. Because once we truly accept who we are—a temporary wave-like extension of universal life energy—we see the world and all sentient and non-sentient beings in a different light. We treat the earth, animals large and small, humans of all color, race, and creed, exactly how we wish to be treated—with acceptance, compassion, and love. These are the three great behaviors that free us from our delusion of separation.

You cannot help but be the wave. You do have karmic free will to behave as if you are not. To do so, however, is to deny your true nature and only prolongs your own personal suffering in this lifetime. So enjoy riding your wave, but understand you have no choice but to return to the sea.

Exercise: Power to Change

We have talked about change numerous times. We should expect it. We are the only ones who can change who and what we are. We are the only ones who can change our circumstances. We talked about it being as simple and as difficult as changing our mindset, our frame of reference. But how do we actually do this? Here is an exercise to get you started:

1. Sit relaxed in an upright position.

2. Clear stress from your body and relax with eyes closed.

3. Visualize what it is you want to change about yourself. Remember you cannot change others—only yourself.

4. Now with the image clearly in your mind, visualize placing a veil of transparent cloth over the image. You can see the image of the old you but it is no longer available to you.

5. On this veil, visualize the new image of yourself. See it clearly in full detail. Absorb the image into your eyes, absorb it into your ears—what does it sound like? What does it feel like? Absorb it into every cell of your body. Absorb it into your mouth, what does it taste like? What are the language and vocabulary of the new image? What is the mindset of the new image?

6. Feel yourself become that image.

7. Behind this veil, drop another transparent veil. From the old you, bring forth all that you want to keep of your present self. Do a thorough examination of all that is great and wonderful about you. If you cannot find anything, you are not trying hard enough. Remove the false image of deficiency and look again.

8. Now you have two veils—that which you desire to keep and that which you desire to be. Pull the two veils together now as one. The image of your former self behind the veils is now disappearing—it is gone.

9. Visualize laying the veils over you now. This is the new you. Feel the veils becoming one with you. Absorbing into your cellular being. Now adapt to the changes and believe it is real and possible.

To Be Reborn

What does it mean to be reborn? Many Christians use the word to mean they have found a new religious direction for their life. Addicts often use the term after they finish a stint in rehab.

Buddhists give a different meaning to the word rebirth. Most people would immediately think of reincarnation or maybe transmigration of the soul. This does involve karmic rebirth, however, that is not the critical interpretation of the word for Buddhists. Rebirth takes place each new moment—there are thousands of rebirths each day. Each second is a new opportunity to see the world and your place in it. Each situation is a new opportunity to practice detachment and compassion. Each time we make a conscious effort to help to relieve the suffering or pain of others; we are reborn again, that very moment.

Change happens and it often happens without us even noticing it. One morning we wake up and the person looking back at us in the mirror somehow looks different than the one who brushed their teeth and washed their face the night before. We are different. Old cells die and slough off; hair grows, turns gray, and falls out. Skin wrinkles despite the expensive miracle cream that promises to maintain our youth. These changes are important, but they are only mile markers of our current existence. Reminders that we came into this life with a task to complete and we are gradually marching toward the end of the time period to complete the task.

Twice today, I heard two different people talk about losing a family member unexpectedly—one was an eight-year old boy who was killed in a freak baseball accident. The father said, "Love your children every day; you never know when it will be the last."

Are you prepared to witness that flash of your life to pass in front of your eyes? It is said in Tibetan Buddhism that upon death we are the one to judge—to judge ourselves as to whether or not this lifetime was successful. We can easily make that assessment at any point to see where we stand before the culminating moment arrives.

Upon what guidelines or standards will you judge? A successful life is NOT one of material wealth, great job, or Harvard education. You will instead measure yourself solely based on how compassionate you were to your fellow man, woman, child, animals, nature, animate and inanimate objects—in short, everything. This is what is important. It does not require wealth, fame, or position to extend a loving hand, word, or smile. It is not so easy when you realize that this means dissolving your anger, greed, ignorance, fear, and hate toward all people at all times without exception.

To be reborn means to take the steps toward compassionate thoughts and behaviors. The opportunity presents itself each moment we live. If you blow it one moment, you have a chance to try it again the next. Once you vow to live a life of compassion, the successful moments will begin to outweigh those when we lapse into our animal mentality. The goal is to get to the point where we no longer make conscious choices to walk the compassionate path, we just do it.

Exercise: The New Me

Take this moment to assess your life up to now. How do you judge its success?

Part Three: Additional Practices

What about yourself will you change and improve? ***When will you do it?***

You never know when your workshop of life will expire. Make the best of it!

Part Three: Additional Practices

Ending is the Beginning

We have been talking about seven critical actions that when practiced in earnest will change your life. On the surface it is easy to say—just let go of old ideas that no longer serve you: old angers, old feelings of being separate and isolated, old feelings of being judged or judging others, or old fears that keep us from reaching our full potential to be happy. We can tell ourselves that we understand holding all these false ideas is not in our best interest. We can vow to let them go. The problem is, it's not that easy.

We develop behavior patterns around those fallacies. The behaviors become habits and then we falsely begin to believe that who we are at our core is the sum total of those behaviors and thoughts. If we shed all that we believe we are, then won't we lose ourselves? Who will we be if not for the identities we built over a lifetime?

Only you can answer this question for yourself. Are your current life patterns causing chaos in your mind? Do they play out in behaviors and attitudes that make you doubt yourself and your abilities? Do you wake up each morning thrilled to face the day or do you feel exhausted before you even get out of bed?

If you are seeking a more peaceful existence within yourself, then take up the challenge of letting go of your attachments to the past and the false image of who you are. Get to know the real you, not the contrived you. It is a natural human response to not want to let go of what we have, what we worked for and built, even when what we have is detrimental to our health and well-being. It is still ours and we want it. We feel that if we let it go, somehow we will lose ourselves. We will cease to exist. This is true but in a good way.

Think of it like this. You are a walking egg. Within the egg are all the nutrients you need for a whole and fulfilling life. The nutrients of acceptance, compassion, and the vital connection of love energy to the universe. All of these are waiting for you to absorb, to use, to become them. Just like the embryo of any species is destined to become whatever the contributing DNA factors are within the shell, so too are we destined to become— eventually—our spiritual energetic, natural DNA.

The shell that surrounds the embryo consists of the false ideas, behaviors, and habits we develop and believe to be who we are. Eventually, our essential self—spiritual being, inner buddha, god energy, grace—will naturally expand and grow in size. Think of the embryo as containing every molecular cell you will ever need or become but it is tightly compacted. As you let the light of truth transform you, the light gently begins to expand the molecules out. You change from a hard, densely compacted ball contained in a shell of old sufferings to something new and expansive. As the light of truth expands the molecules outward you become lighter, more airy and free, better able to see the world/life from a different aspect—outside of the confining false shell that falls away. Our ever-expanding self now has the ability to touch others, to surround them in hope, understanding, support, and compassionate care.

When we are free of our false shell, there are no limits to our peace and happiness. We are free to choose—yes choose—the full life we what to live. Free to choose a life of peace, joy, and contentment. Rather than mourning the loss of who you were, see the transformation as a growth to new heights, reaching the full potential of who you really are.

Your DNA strands are acceptance, compassion, and love. Acceptance—that all is as it should be for this moment in time for all those involved, to learn whatever it is you need to learn, to expand beyond your self-created shell. Compassion—to understand, to nurture yourself and others through this expansion process. We all have our own personal set of growth instructions based on our karmically accumulated past lives and actions during this lifetime. We need the compassion and support of others—and ourselves for ourselves—to be able to have the courage to stay with the process and not give up. The final DNA strand is love—the connecting universal life energy—this is the breath that sustains us. It is the air we breathe. It is the nucleus of the molecule. Love—me—you—life—energy—peace, it is all the same. It is you in your purest form. You simply need to acknowledge it. Instead of mourning the loss of your accumulated old thoughts and behaviors, celebrate the coming home to the real life you are intended to live. It is your birth right. It is in your DNA to be peace. If you are peace, then how can you live in anything else? Claim your birthright now, it is available to you. Be your peace and best wishes for a rapid expansion.

Glossary

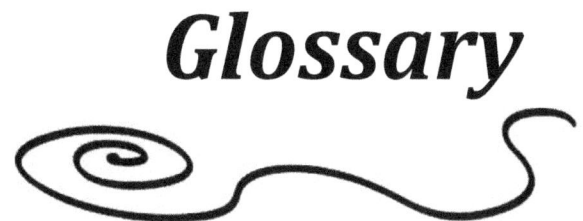

Buddha-nature

Buddha-nature is the concept that all sentient beings are born with all the qualities of the Buddha. The qualities may not be exhibited at the present time, but they will be in the *future once the person gains the ability to eliminate all suffering. Just a few of the qualities include abolishment of greed, abolishment of attachment and ego, and the presence of total peace and enlightenment. Physical pain can never be completely avoided, but mental and emotional suffering that result from physical pain can be eliminated.

Bodhisattva

Enlightened beings who have agreed to come back into body to help others end their suffering. Also an ordinary person who diligently practices the teachings of the Buddha and hold as their primary purpose in life, to live in total compassion for others.

Chakras

There are seven major energy centers or openings in the body through which we are energetically connected to the universe. Each center has a different function in the body, mind, and emotions. If one or more of the openings are energetically blocked or closed, illness can result. Locations of the chakras are shown in the following table, moving from the base of the body to the head.

When a person has problems in the emotion/mental areas, the associated chakra begins to close down. The parts of the body that are near the chakra become sluggish. With long-term emotional and mental suffering, the parts of the body can become diseased and cease to function. Additional information on chakras can be found on numerous web sites.

#	Name	Location	Emotional/Mental Reflections	Color
1	Root	Base of the spine, in the tailbone region	Our basic material needs for survival	Red
2	Sacral	Lower abdomen, about 2 inches below the navel	Child-like openness, creativity, family relationships, and sexuality	Orange
3	Solar Plexus	Abdomen about 1 inch above the	The center of the body, balance, self-worth, self-confidence, and career	Yellow

#	Name	Location	Emotional/Mental Reflections	Color
		navel		
4	Heart	Center of the chest, between the breasts	Our ability to love, feel joy, happiness, connectedness with others, and peace	Green
5	Throat	Base of the throat	Our ability to clearly speak our truth and feelings	Blue
6	Third Eye	Between the eye brows	Intuition, wisdom, ability to think clearly and make decisions	Indigo
7	Crown	At the crown or top of the head	Our ability to be fully connected energetically to the universe or a person's personal spirituality	White

How to use the Buddhist tools of "The Four Noble Truths," "Six Perfections," and the "Eightfold Path"

The Four Noble Truths state that life is full of suffering, but if you determine the cause of the suffering, it can be eliminated. Typically, the vast majority of suffering results from not following the Six Perfections or the Eightfold Path. If you understand how to use these tools, then it is easy to identify where you are making mistakes and correct the situation.

For example, it is natural to interpret situations that we find ourselves in through a filter distorted by our past experiences. Quite often this leads us to misinterpret other people's meanings and intentions, and consequently conflict arises. By using the Eightfold Path first principle of Right View, we remove the filter and see the situation from a non-biased point of view. This permits us to see the situation for what it really is.

- A man we do not know walks our direction in the parking lot of a grocery store.

- We immediately think that the person looks scruffy and is going to beg for money.

- Our defenses and maybe our anxiety level rises. We feel scared and hostile.

- He then gets into a car parked next to ours and greets us with a smile saying, "Good Morning to you!" and drives away.

The unfiltered situation is that a man was walking in the parking lot. Everything else was made up as a result of our filter of fear.

The following Buddhist interpretations come from the Basic Teachings of Buddhism guidebook published by Rissho Kosei-kai International of North America (RKINA) (2013).

Eightfold Path

The word *"right"* means to be in harmony with the Buddha's Teaching of Universal Truth *(Dharma)*. It involves looking at things from a viewpoint that is not self-centered, but includes care for others. A viewpoint that comes from a clear, open, and flexible mind that takes into account other perspectives and other possibilities.

1. Right View: Abandon self-centered ways and see situations as they really are.

2. Right Thought: Think from a higher standard and point of view. Eliminate greediness, resentment, and evil-mindedness. Think with a generous mind.

3. Right Speech: In your speech, be compassionate, empathetic, and tolerant.

4. Right Action: Act with integrity in all you do.

5. Right Livelihood: Obtain the necessities of life through a vocation that is useful to society and beneficial to a person's mental, emotional, and physical health.

6. Right Endeavor: Always do good deeds and apply yourself diligently in carrying out the teachings.

7. Right Mindfulness: Be mindful and remain in the present moment without prejudice or creating stories from ignorance.

8. Right Concentration: Practice quieting the mind and developing the ability to single-pointedly focus the mind so as to not to become agitated by any change of circumstances. (RKINA 19)

Enlightenment

Enlightenment is a state of perfect knowledge or wisdom, combined with infinite compassion. Knowledge in this case means that one understands the reality of the truth of all existence: we are all one, everything that occurs is based on cause and effect, and everything changes. With this total understanding and practice, we are able to extinguish the suffering in our life.

Four Noble Truths

Truth of Suffering *Buddha saw birth, sickness, old age, and death as normal suffering*	**Truth of Cause** *Twelve-link chain of causation-dependent origination*
First step is to acknowledge the suffering, which can be spiritual, physical, mental, economic, or emotional.	Second step is to investigate the specific and deep cause of suffering. Nothing exists in isolation, everything has a cause.
Truth of Extinction	**Truth of the Path (end suffering)** *Guidelines for action*
Third step is knowing that there is a tranquil state, without suffering, whether it be spiritual, physical, mental, economic, or emotional.	Fourth step is practicing the appropriate teaching to extinguishing suffering: –The Eightfold Path –The Six Perfections

(RKINA 7)

Six Perfections/Paramitas

1. Donation (generosity): Be generous with your time, attention, and wealth. Use them to sincerely serve the community and other people.

2. Ethical Guidelines (keeping the precepts or following the teachings): Be ethical, humble, and disciplined.

3. Forbearance (patience): Be patient with yourself and others, remove irritability.

4. Effort (diligence): Endeavor constantly and give your full effort at all times.

5. Meditation: Be calm and clear your mind.

6. Wisdom: Remove prejudice and selfish thinking through increased awareness and experience. (RKINA 22)

Three Treasures

Refuge means that a person should find comfort, safety, and protection in each of the Three Treasures.

1. Take refuge in the Buddha.

    Buddha is a great treasure because of the teachings and role modeling he provided to all.

2. Take refuge in the Dharma.

    Dharma is another word for the teachings of Shakyamuni Buddha.

3. Take refuge in the Sangha.

    The Sanskrit word *sangha* means "an intimate and faithful group consisting of many believers." It is difficult to practice the teachings in isolation. It much easier to practice with a community of believers that support each other. For this reason, the Buddha considered the sangha to be the most important of the Three Treasures. (RKINA 1)

The Ten Commandments from the Christian Bible

1. You shall have no other gods before Me.

2. You shall not make idols.

3. You shall not take the name of the Lord your God in vain.

4. Remember the Sabbath day, to keep it holy.

5. Honor your father and your mother.

6. You shall not murder.

7. You shall not commit adultery.

8. You shall not steal.

9. You shall not bear false witness against your neighbor.

10. You shall not covet your neighbor's wife…or anything that is your neighbor's.

Bibliography

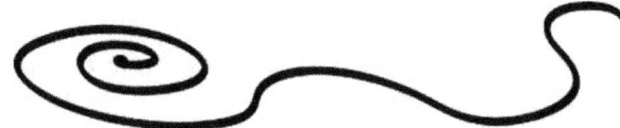

Allport, Gordon W., *The Nature of Prejudice: 25th Anniversary Edition.* New York: Perseus Books Publishing, LLC, 1979. Print

Brach, PhD, Tara, *Radical Acceptance: Embracing Your Life with the Heart of a Buddha.* New York: Bantam Books, 2003. Print

Braden, Gregg, *The Divine Matrix: Bridging Time, Space, Miracles, and Belief.* Carlsbad, CA: Hay House Publishing, 2008. Print

Blanton, Brad, *Radical Parenting: Seven Steps to a Functional Family in a Dysfunctional World.* Stanley, VA: Sparrowhawk Publications, 2004. Print

Carter, Les, *The Anger Trap: Free Yourself from the Frustrations that Sabotage Your Life.* New York: John Wiley & Sons, 2004. Print

Chopra, Deepak, *The Seven Spiritual Laws of Success: A Practical Guide to the Fulfillment of Your Dreams.* San Rafael, CA: Publishers Group West, 1994. Print

Chopra, Deepak, *The Way of the Wizard: Twenty Spiritual Lessons for Creating the Life You Want.* New York: Harmony Books, 1995. Print

Hanh, Thich Nhat, *Anger: Wisdom for Cooling the Flames.* New York: Riverhead Trade, 2002. Print

Hill, Charles W.L., *Global Business.* 7th ed New York: McGraw-Hill Irwin, 2011. Print

Ianniello, Nick, "Dealing with the Effect of Fear Anxieties," *The Appalachian.* October 31, 2006. Print

Jeffers PhD, Susan, *Feel the Fear and Beyond.* New York: Ballantine Publish Group, 1998. Print

Lama, Dalai XIV, *The Art of Happiness: A Handbook for Living.* New York: Riverhead Books, 1998. Print

Mullins, George A., *Raising Up Bodhisattvas in the Modern Ages.* Tokyo: Kosei Publishing, 2002. Print

National Geographic, "Origins of the Universe—An Expanding World," National Geographic Website, http://science.nationalgeographic.com/science/space/universe/origins-universe-article October 6, 2014.Digital.

Niwano, Kosho, *The Buddha in Everyone's Heart: Seeking the World of the Lotus Sutra.* Tokyo: Kosei Publishing, 2013. Print

Niwano, Nikkyo, *Buddhism for Everyday Life: Memorable Dharma Messages from a Long Spiritual Journey.* Tokyo: Kosei Publishing, 2011. Print

Niwano, Nikkyo, *Buddhism for Today: A Modern Interpretation of the Threefold Lotus Sutra.* Tokyo: Kosei Publishing, 1976. Print

Ruiz, Don Miguel, *The Four Agreements: A Practical Guide to Personal Freedom.* San Rafael CA: Amber-Allen Publishing,1997.

Rissho Kosei-kai International of North America (RKINA), *Guide to the Basic Teachings.* Los Angeles, CA, 2013. Print

Tulkin, Tarthang, ed, *Reflections of the Mind: Western Psychology Meets Tibetan Buddhism.* Emeryville, CA: Dharma Publishing, 1975. Print

Veenestra, Rene, Siegwart Lindenbert, Andrea F. De Winter, Albertine J. Oldehinkel, Frank C. Verhulst, and Johan Ormel, "Bullying and Victimization in Elementary Schools: A Comparison of Bullies, Victims, Bully/Victims, and Uninvolved Preadolescents, "*Developmental Psychology*, Vol 41.4 (2005): 672-682. Print

Walsh, Roger, *Essential Spirituality: The 7 Central Practices to Awaken Heart and Mind.* New York: John Wiley & Sons, 1999. Print

About the Author

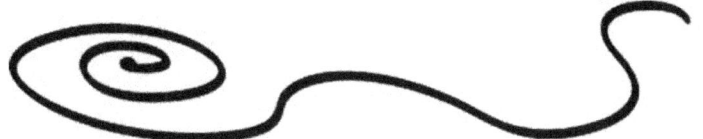

The time Reverend Dr. Perri spends as the spiritual leader and director of the Rissho Kosei-kai Dharma Center of Dayton is precious and rewarding. Using her training as a Buddhist Dharma Teacher and ordained interfaith minister, she offers a safe place for people of all faiths to come, learn about their true inner selves, and heal.

Jane Perri, Ph.D, DHT, OUnI has extensive experience as an organizational consultant guiding businesses and industry to develop a more effective and congenial workplace.

She is also an associate professor at the Oregon Institute of Technology, Klamath Falls, OR, where she is the Program Director for the online Sleep Health programs and teaches in the Management Department.

Go to **www.CriticalActionsWorkbook.com** to find out about workshops and speaking engagements to help bring the healing message of this book to life.

www.ingramcontent.com/pod-product-compliance
Lightning Source LLC
Chambersburg PA
CBHW080555090426
42735CB00016B/3239